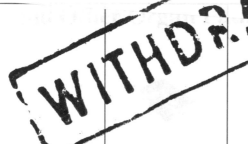

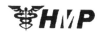

The Haworth Medical Press®
An Imprint of The Haworth Press, Inc.

Enteroviral and Toxin Mediated Myalgic Encephalomyelitis/ Chronic Fatigue Syndrome and Other Organ Pathologies

THE HAWORTH MEDICAL PRESS®
Chronic Fatigue Syndrome, Fibromyalgia Syndrome, and Myalgic Encephalomyelitis

Roberto Patarca-Montero, MD, PhD
Senior Editor

Enteroviral and Toxin Mediated Myalgic Encephalomyelitis/ Chronic Fatigue Syndrome and Other Organ Pathologies

John Richardson, MB, BS

The Haworth Medical Press®
An Imprint of The Haworth Press, Inc.
New York • London • Oxford

Published by

The Haworth Medical Press®, an imprint of The Haworth Press, Inc., 10 Alice Street, Binghamton, NY 13904-1580

Medicine is an ever-changing science. As new research and clinical experience broaden our knowledge, changes in treatment and drug therapy are required. While many suggestions for drug usages or treatment regimens are made herein, the book is intended for educational purposes only, and the author, editor, and publisher do not accept liability in the event of negative consequences incurred as a result of information presented in this book. We do not claim that this information is necessarily accurate by the rigid scientific standard applied for medical proof, and therefore make no warranty, expressed or implied, with respect to the material herein contained. Therefore the patient is urged to check the product information sheet included in the package of each drug he or she plans to administer to be certain the protocol followed is not in conflict with the manufacturer's inserts. When a discrepancy arises between these inserts and information in this book, the physician is encouraged to use his or her best professional judgment.

Cover design by Jennifer M. Gaska.

Library of Congress Cataloging-in-Publication Data

Richardson, John, 1915-
    Enteroviral and toxin mediated myalgic encephalomyelitis/chronic fatigue syndrome and other organ pathologies / John Richardson.
        p. cm.
    Includes bibliographical references and index.
    ISBN 0-7890-1127-1 (alk. paper)—ISBN 0-7890-1128-X (alk. paper)
    1. Virus diseases—Complications. 2. Myalgic encephalomyelitis—Etiology. 3. Chronic fatigue syndrome—Etiology. 4. Host-virus relationships. I. Title.

RC114.5 .R53 2001
616´.0194—dc21
                                                                                                00-054146

CONTENTS

ABOUT THE AUTHOR

Dr. John Richardson, MB, BS, has been a family practitioner since 1953. He earned his medical degree from Newcastle upon Tyne University where he became a Founder Member of the Department of Family Medicine and a tutor in family medicine for four decades. Dr. Richardson was recognized as a General Practitioner Obstetrician at the Princess Mary Maternity Hospital. He delivered more than 5,000 babies and undertook four decades of research into primary infertility.

Dr. Richardson is a Founder Member of the Newcastle Research Group, as well as a member of the Melvin Ramsey Society, the Environmental Medicine Association, and other medical research organizations. He has published a number of articles, including pioneering work on drug-food interactions and effects of pesticide poisoning. He has served as a Regional Medical Officer for the Ministry of Health, as a Senior Police Surgeon, and as a member of the Police Surgeon's Advisory Panel. He served as Chairman of the 1989 Cambridge Symposium on the Clinical and Scientific Basis of Myalgic Encephalomyelitis.

Foreword

It is uncommon to find one who has devoted half a century of his professional life to one subject. John Richardson has done just that, starting with a clinical interest in the consequences of enteroviral infections, and continuing on to study patients with fatigue syndromes of other etiologies. In the outskirts of Newcastle where he works, his semirural practice also has patients with organophosphorus (OP) poisoning as a consequence of sheep "dipping" with OP agents. This fact has led to the study of many fatigue patients with exposure to other toxins.

John Richardson has seen large numbers of his own patients with the consequences of persistent enteroviral infections, and his general practice has had many more referred to him. In this book are set out some of the consequences not previously recognized, such as peritoneal mesothelioma and birth defects as well as the virus-associated fatigue syndromes, usually called myalgic encephalomyelitis or ME. Though strictly the term ME should be limited to chronic fatigue syndromes associated with specific virus infections, he has chosen to use the older meaning, what is more commonly called CFS or chronic fatigue syndrome today. In the United Kingdom fatigue syndromes are most commonly associated with persistent enteroviral infection, and the studies in the community of John Richardson and others lead one to believe that it is probably as common in other temperate climes. In the United States it is not as well appreciated, although Western Europe and Canada have largely accepted such an association. In recent years HIV has become a common cause of fatigue syndromes in the United States, but Richardson's experience has included many hundreds of fatigue patients associated with enteroviruses, and very few with HIV.

The studies in this book involve many collaborators, as John is very good at bullying, cajoling, and encouraging others to help him in the laboratory and hospital investigation of his patients. The association of investigation and clinical presentation has been a very important study to him, and they are presented here for your enlightenment.

I was caught up in John Richardson's clinical studies about twenty years ago and have benefited from the experience. From him I have learned of family associations of viruses and fatigue syndromes, of the importance of OP poisoning in the production of permanent neurological damage accompanied by fatigue syndromes, and a unique, bizarre presentation of enteroviral infection. I have learned much from him, not only in the clinical and scientific results, but also in the value of a scientist in general practice, seeing the interactions of family, genetics, and environment in the presentation and development of disease. I hope that the reader enjoys the experience also.

James F. Mowbray
Emeritus Professor of Immunopathology
Imperial College School of Medicine at St. Mary's, London

Introduction

Compiling an introduction to a book forty years after the events that initiated the work is a challenge. Varied experiences in medicine at varying levels, both at home and abroad, produced in my mind an aphorism that is still relevant. It applies after the completion of a piece of research, perhaps after giving a lecture in which the results are outlined, or even when reading the results of the work of others in printed articles. The end result is the aphorism "more questions than answers." This remains the same today, and hopefully the chapters of this book will stimulate further thought and work, with "some answers and more questions." Although my research has been done in a semirural practice setting, I must pay tribute to my many colleagues in various laboratories and hospital departments, for without their cooperation the work could not have been done. The names are too numerous to mention and include many local to my practice in the northeast of England and others elsewhere in the United Kingdom and abroad.

I spent quite a number of years in hospital work with experience in general medicine, surgery, cardiology, neurology, pediatrics, obstetrics, and pathology. All of this furnished a good background for further work in community medicine.

That much has changed in the past forty years is obvious. This applies to the environment and to changing patterns of illness. Forty years ago, as a senior house orderly in a local hospital, I admitted a young man in his twenties with dyspnea, headache, and general limb pains. He had collapsed, and an electrocardiogram (ECG) was aberrant but not diagnostic of an infarct. Sadly, he died, and at autopsy his heart was patchy and inflamed with a softened left ventricle, but the coronary arteries were quite patent and healthy. The pathologist of the day stated that the young man had a myocardial infarct, and the clot had lysed. I was never happy about this diagnosis, and the experience remained with me. Since then papers have been published referring to the possibility that viruses are agents in the initiation of myocardial infarction as well as myocarditis. Other members of this man's family had been ill with some odd sort of viral illness, but I could not investigate. It was apparent to me that in the hospital setting I was remote from the families, and though I could "take a history," it did not give me the opportunity to have an integral part in community life.

In addition, in the hospital setting specialization was becoming more than ever the order of the day. This had obvious benefits but also quite serious limitations. Thus I felt that I was seeing a single patient in an isolated setting and often felt limited in having to deal only with the immediate presenting illness. In contrast, it was apparent to me that the true family doctor could relate patient to family, family to community, and present illness to past health both acute or sequential, as well as to familial illness either by contagion or genetics.

For these reasons, I decided to practice in family medicine. I moved to an old established practice in Blaydon and set up a surgery in nearby Ryton. This made a practice of three partners serving around 6,000 patients, which steadily increased. The area has changed but is still more or less rural and has the advantage of a population with strong family ties going back for generations in some cases. This became the ideal situation for studying sequential illness in both individuals and families. Other colleagues became involved in the work, and we subsequently formed what is now known as the Newcastle Research Group (NRG). This group has attracted attention from researchers around the world and has become a forum for annual international conferences.

Shortly after entering this practice, I was called to see a Scottish patient and learned his history. He had come home from the war in 1946 and developed headache and vertigo while out shopping with his wife. Later he developed a rash on his trunk, upper limbs, and neck. The previous doctor, a sagacious man of long experience, wrote in his notes, "It looks like rubella but it is not rubella." He also found that after this illness the patient developed a heart murmur. The doctor sent him to a hospital, but nothing definitive came of it. He was off work for two years. A year later, in 1949, he had a further episode identical to the first. He was again referred to a hospital but was told that it was "mostly his nerves." In 1955 he was quite ill, and I found marked evidence of congestive failure with a very abnormal ECG. Moreover, he had serological evidence of previous coxsackie B group 4 infection. My colleague, Dr. H. A. Dewar, saw him with me and agreed that he had clinical signs of cardiomyopathy. He was sustained for six years but died in 1961, and the postmortem did show a cardiomyopathy. These and other events, referred to in subsequent chapters, were the means of stimulating my interest in postviral-mediated syndromes.

For a long while, though the varying dicta that one is taught influenced my thinking and approach, it became clear that in many cases subsequent illnesses did not fit into the patterns expected. Various illnesses that would be considered unrelated to past history emerged and were treated as new and separate entities. By the time I was in family medicine and able to observe families and individual patients, the evidence pointed to the fact that the dicta were wrong. The dicta pointed to and were concerned with the disease, whereas my approach has veered ever more strongly toward the patient—and a "holistic" approach.

This did not lead to simplification, however, yet it caused me to think more deeply and question my whole approach to "illness," as being not an entity in itself but something that was active and aberrant in the patient.

A few simple correlates have emerged:

1. Viruses and bacteria have been with us a long time.
2. Our lifestyle has changed over the years, for both good and ill. For good, as general nourishment and welfare has improved; for ill in that we expose ourselves to more environmental pollution and many other self-inflicted insults, such as smoking, alcohol, drugs, etc.
3. However, it has been brought home to me that some can go on smoking into their seventies and do not seem to suffer. Others drink or eat foolishly, yet survive. Of all the millions who smoke, only a small minority die of bronchogenic carcinoma, which the "public" think of as the only serious effect. Again, in the period when tuberculosis (TB) was not treated by modern antituberculous therapy, most people became Mantoux positive by their school years. In these people, though a severe and chronic sequence of illness could ensue, it occurred only in a minority, and the others developed their own immunity. This undoubtedly applied to other bacterial and

viral infections to which natural immunity developed, such as smallpox, poliomyelitis, etc.

Thus we have survived these challenges. Indeed it became a form of treatment to inoculate patients with attenuated Tubercle bacilli in some cases of malignant disease as a means of stimulating the immune system. Smallpox was eradicated by vaccination and not by antibiotics, which perhaps should have caused us to think more than we have done. Calmette-Guérin bacillus followed the same pattern of vaccination for prevention, not of infection, but of succumbing to the disease. In this category we could place diphtheria, pertussis, tetanus, typhoid, polio, yellow fever, cholera, and hepatitis B, among others.

In the case of malaria, the control of the intermediate host, as well as the use of antimalarial drugs, has been employed with some success, but so-called resistant strains have emerged, showing that this is not as effective as immunization. These are only examples of efforts at disease control.

It is apparent from these examples, however, that stimulation of the immune system by immunization has been most effective and may have a lifetime effect. However, another assumption was, and still is, made that Pasteur "invented" immunization.

The fact is that nature has been practicing immunization, and without it the species might have become extinct long ago. Another assumption that I feel has been carried too far is the concept that there are organisms which are by nature "virulent" and some which by their intrinsic nature are "nonpathogenic." It would appear, however, that all organisms given certain conditions can be pathogenic; thus the observation of *virulence de passage* is true, and by this means organisms develop species virulence.

Certain plagues such as bubonic plague, typhus, and typhoid, just to mention three, have affected humanity down the centuries and, as there was no general natural immunity, the results were devastating. With the advent of antibiotics we have changed the course of events somewhat; certainly in the case of TB, etc., those who do develop the disease due to lack of effective immune control can be "cured" by antibiotic therapy.

However, we have extended antibiotic therapy to a whole range of infectious conditions, and patients now almost universally expect any infection to be treated with antibiotics. I would suggest that by such treatment we have deprived the immune system of its challenge, and the ability to respond has thereby been decreased.

In a survey of cases over a five-year period, I have annotated those with viral and those with obvious bacterial etiology. Thirty years ago most "serious" cases were bacterial; today, while serious bacterial cases still occur, the number of cases that are viral far outnumber them. In this analysis, whereas in the 1950s, 80 percent of cases were bacterial and 20 percent were viral, this is now simply reversed. Perhaps venereal disease is a pertinent example. The bacterial forms have proved treatable and so are lightly esteemed, but the present prospect of HIV and AIDS constitutes a much more formidable problem. Unlike the bacterial forms, they are so much more severe and lethal.

We can also consider the difference between mice and humans as models. In their natural habitat mice do not smoke, etc.—but humans do not live in soil, and maybe the pollutants of soil affect mice more adversely than humans. However, it is possible to expose mice as models to the varying conditions that affect us and condition them or other mammals in precisely the same way. Then extrapolation can occur, and it is possible to look at disease processes in either the conditioned mice or humans and compare them. For us, however, an additional factor in the spread of disease is the advent of easy travel by road, sea, and air. Also, convenient water supplies, which depend on reservoirs in developed countries, have created a new source of potential infection. As we travel, so do birds, and the latter congregate at reservoirs and thus use our water supply. Many viruses have been recovered from the cloacae of birds and also from reservoir water. Thus we no longer live a cloistered life and are subject to the possibility of both familiar and hitherto unfamiliar infections. It is interesting that the seasonal outbreaks of viruses coincide with the seasonal movements of birds.

Compounding the problem is the matter of immunosuppression. Genetic considerations exist, for, despite viruses and insults from chemical agents such as cigarette smoke or pollution from insecticides and so on (which are foolishly thought to be "lethal" to "lower forms of life" but "harmless" to us as a "higher form of life"), only a proportion of people appear to have disease as a result, as has been shown in the mouse model. It is clearly too much to ask that we should all know our genetic composition and to what we might succumb. We are not bred in such pure strains as the animal models.

This brief summary shows that we are presently not dealing with transient illnesses nor yet with a single epidemic" such as the Black Death. It would appear wise to consider in more detail the integration and functioning of the immune system, its relationship to invasive disease, and the means whereby it can be rendered more fully competent. It should be obvious that we have survived by this means and not by medicine, albeit the latter has its place.

It would be wise to try to elucidate the means whereby the host has successfully dealt with these challenges. It may prove to be more rewarding than the search for antiviral agents themselves, especially if we learn the lesson that the antibiotic era may be able to teach us.

Thus, the immunological approach to the control of disease would appear to be the most effective and rational. It would involve both immunization and also ways of augmenting the effects of the immune system in the event of challenge and, equally important, avoiding anything organic or inorganic that would suppress the autoimmune system. Already this is being pursued both at home and abroad and will have more lasting effects than the development of antibiotics or antiviral agents. By the latter methods we may shorten, eliminate, or alter the acute phase of an illness, yet, as shown earlier, we may diminish the immune response, which would not be to our advantage for subsequent infection. I would soberly suggest that we have entered the "viral age of disease."

Madsen (1934), in his foreword to Sylvest's monograph *Epidemic Myalgia—Bornholm Disease,* makes the observation that "present day medical research tends to gravitate to hospital and laboratory but the work of Dr. Sylvest shows that there nevertheless exists a vast field of clinical investigation, open to those general practitioners who possess an independent and unbiased power of observation of the variegated pictures of illness." I wish to be one such and after thirty-six years also make some observations, recognizing however that the interpretation I place on them may or may not ultimately prove to be correct.

We function within the concepts instilled in us by our teachers, and these concepts basically are the teachers' interpretations of observations. The observations may be correct but the interpretations incorrect. It is the latter I have had to challenge, while going back to pure observation itself has been helpful. The following sections describe some of my challenges.

SAPROPHYTIC VERSUS PATHOGENIC

I now take a simple view and say that all is saprophytic providing it remains in territory where it can be utilized by host activity. Of course we call this symbiosis, but then we go on to restrict, modify, or complicate the issue. *E. coli* function well in the gastrointestinal (GI) tract but cannot find a home or useful occupation in the genitourinary (GU) tract. The flora in the GI tract absorb some of our food and in turn give off a residue that is metabolized and absorbed as part of our vitamin B complex. In the GU tract, this symbiosis does not apply, and therefore the same *E. coli* would be pathogenic. Thus it is the host that determines whether an organism is pathogenic (adverse) or saprophytic (useful).

I believe this applies right across the board to food, bacteria, viruses, prions, etc. This idea is reflected in the function of the herbivore, which is able to convert plant protein, etc., into animal protein whereas carnivores are unable to do the same. This ranges from elephant to mouse—the gut length in herbivores is thirty-three times longer than the spinal cord, whereas the carnivore has a gut length only seven times the length of its spinal cord. It is not the protein that is deficient but the mechanism to process and alter that protein. I believe this idea must be applied in the recognition, absorption, manipulation, and utilization of all elements, of which so-called food is only one. Moreover, it must also apply to every group of cells in the body; i.e., the product processed by the GI tract then becomes a "coded" prototype that would be "recognized" and acceptable in some way to some, if not all, cellular substrates for useful incorporation.

The failure of this holistic mechanism with its varying ramifications is, to my mind, the chief cause of disease. This may be due to some intrinsic failure to "recognize and absorb" only that which is useful; or conversely, not to recognize and reject that which may be potentially harmful or, as we term it, pathogenic. This shifts the responsibility for pathogenicity more to the host cell. I am aware, of course, that some elements are "poisonous" in their own right, and I do not exclude the "mental selection" by the host of what may be known to be compatible with its own welfare, e.g., nicotine. Of course, that is another matter not in the scope of this study.

ARE THERE "NEW" VIRUSES OR BACTERIA?

My own reading would lead me to consider that there are no new viruses or bacteria. Do they "mutate"? Again, my reasoning would now say "No." Pasteur's work and observations are valid and good, but the construction we place on them and on other work should be guarded. He did coin the term *resistance de passage,* which, in my opinion, meant a species caused an organism to mutate to be more "acceptable" to it as a host and therefore less acceptable to any other species, including humans.

It has been stated that a virus cannot proliferate in a noncellular medium, and the inference is drawn that in a cellular medium, it takes over the host mechanism to reproduce itself. I consider that the cell reproduces the virus and not vice versa. Perhaps the fact that the host cell can now be shown to reproduce virions or prions, which have no nucleus and are purely protein, should lead us to discard this concept. Again the observation that viruses are reproduced in cell lines is correct, but the construction put upon it is incorrect, to my mind. It is the host that is the active agent and pathologically reproduces virus or virus protein within its membrane to its own destruction or until the sick cell syndrome develops as a prelude to cell death or malignancy. It is well to remember that malignant cells are in reality belonging to the host albeit reduced to pleomorphic abnormal forms, which the host sometimes then treats as embryogenic and will "coat," in some cases with human chorionic gonadotrophin (HCG), thus presenting a problem for the immune system.

THE "MUTATION THEORY"

I have no doubt about the observations, but different interpretations can be made. Just as the elephant may absorb and alter protein to suit basic cellular requirements, and this protein goes on to more sophisticated processing later prior to incorporation, so too viral protein is being absorbed, perhaps continuously or in seasonal spreads, and is also being processed by the host, which may be bird, animal, or human. This is symbiosis in a general way. The protein—virus in this case—is manipulated by its immediate host and might be "changed" like any other ingested element, to be incorporated into host tissue. This we might call virus species mutation. However, from the study of 300 to 400 families in my series, it can easily be shown that there is not only "species" mutation but "familial" mutation; i.e., species within species.

The facts are that in over 300 families, where one member has been ill with a presumed viral illness, other members of the family have had equally high titers of the same virus, without any illness. In many families this has been repeated over a few years, and eventually another member succumbs to the same virus, but having a titer no higher than that previously recorded. It is merely a matter of observation that the initial titer recorded may not be the highest nor represent the first serological encounter of host with virus.

Could this fact validate the concept of familial mutation? During the passage of virus through other previously affected members, does the host "change"—i.e., "mutate"—the virus so that it is more readily accepted by another host of similar genetic strain within the family? I believe we must think along these lines or just adopt the general theory that family members became ill because their "resistance was low" or that they had contracted "another virus," etc.

This raises interesting challenges, for so far we have considered the possibility of the host mutating a virus to the disadvantage of a future host. Of course, we have models that show the opposite to be true. Mainly this mutation applies to passage through different species, so that virulence is lost for one species at the expense of another. However, immunization per se can occur within a species, and this is shown in the families studied, in that in only about 10 percent of families did further members become ill.

The question then is not that of the virulence of the virus, for that was established by an illness, nor was it "cross immunization," for no blood, sera, etc. were involved, and only the virus itself was "shared." Moreover, in some families the same member was ill time after time, with identical serological titers of the same virus, showing perhaps the persistence of a virus with perhaps "family species mutation." In another family a different member became ill later. But again this only occurred in about 10 percent of the families with high titers who were studied. This suggests that immunization had occurred in the other members who exhibited high titers and for this reason maybe the sera of such patients would contain an adequate amount of a neutralizing antibody fraction that would be specific for that viral strain. Obviously this would not be likely to apply to anyone who had died.

Assuming these ideas to be reasonable would justify the concept of using immunoglobulin (IgG) from "immune" family members as a means of treatment by "immunization." This I would consider to be active immunization. However, on the same grounds, I think we have to recognize that there is "autoimmunization," when a person, maybe in the same family, reacts by producing adequate antibodies to a virus to which another member has succumbed; this will protect that member at that time. If the original host harbors the virus and goes on mutating it, then it can become a fresh challenge to any contact, but only 10 percent appear to fail in antibody response and actually become ill later. The mechanisms, of course, are intricate and range from serological or lymphocytic mechanisms to intracellular lymphokines and their associated enzymes. This is for future generations of laboratory workers to investigate. However, at the moment, in certain cases treatment with IgG has been successful as judged by patient response.

For the present, perhaps it is enough to call into question our concepts, to build on what may be perceived as constructive and not as hitherto restrictive, and to regard the host and environment more as a whole. This also may be of particular interest in considering the enteroviruses. The GI tract is extremely sophisticated, from its villi to the Peyer's patches. The lung may breathe, the heart may beat, but the gut is involved in biochemical selection far beyond our understanding. In addition, the brain with its own blood-brain barrier, normally never encountering a lymphocyte, governing all, yet functioning in splendid isolation, is still nourished by what is absorbed in the GI tract. We have subjected the organisms to a great deal of study, which is fine, but if the survival and health of the host depends on host activity, then we should study this in more detail and perhaps learn lessons on the way in which we may apply such activity in therapy.

Finally, in the concept of therapeutics I would like us to clarify our thoughts a little. I find that often it is not realized that treatment is merely symptomatic as opposed to cure, when so often this is the case. The old idiom, *sublata causa tollitur effectus* (remove the cause and the effect will cease), applies more strongly than ever as we now tend to be satisfied by control as opposed to true cure. This may be illustrated for our purpose by two areas only; the central nervous system (CNS) and the cardiovascular system. To illustrate the latter, I have a young man in his second decade with a viral myocarditis and a resultant toxic Wenckebach phenomenon and dysrythmia. He is "controlled" at the moment by class 1 antidysrythmics together with a beta-blocker and Xameterol. It should be plain that this is not a cure, and the aim should be "to remove the cause so that the effect should cease."

Referring to CNS control, so much discussion centers on the use of antidepressants in the syndrome of myalgic encephalomyelitis (ME), when once more we should recognize that they are only symptomatic treatments as are the cardiac antidysrythmic drugs. Perhaps, if we more correctly assessed what we were doing and thus accepted the limitations of treating the effect, we might then be more willing to address ourselves to finding and then treating the cause. A diagnosis of appendicitis is a diagnosis of effect, operation certainly removing both effect and organ, which in this case is superficial. However, the same rationale cannot be applied to, say, the kidney, pancreas, or any other so-called vital organ.

In diffuse disease the treatment of diffuse effects is much more difficult, and a patient with many complaints may be wearisome to us, unless we are very fortunate in defining the root "cause." Its elimination if possible, resulting in restored health, delights the doctor as much as the patient. I would be the first to admit that this is a counsel of perfection, which I rarely achieve, but I think it is good to train our minds to think in this direction, for it is not only the counsel of perfection for cure, but would certainly also be the council of perfection for prevention. It is not the elimination of viruses we should be thinking of; the "cause" in this field is the failure of the host to recognize and reject. To treat the cause we must first recognize it, and in so doing we may make plain the way in which the host can help itself.

This, of course, would apply directly to the transmission of disease as seen in, for example, HIV virus, as well as diseases caused by cigarette smoking, etc. It is obvious that the subject is not gilded with glamour to either the general public or the doctor; nor would it make news, like a heart transplant. It would need a new type of discipline—human responsibilities rather than human rights—and I suspect it would not be so popular. Nevertheless, it is fair to say we do not live or suffer in isolation, for the smoker passes on the noxious fumes to others, the blood donor gives whatever his or her blood may contain, and the recipient receives for good or ill. The donor is responsible. In this way we manipulate our environment with or without careful thought or consideration, affecting ourselves and then one another. That this does have consequences which are far reaching and often more potent than drugs should perhaps cause us to consider what it may teach us in both therapeutic and preventive medicine.

ASSESSING EPIDEMIOLOGICAL STUDIES

Finally, we may have to assess what we are logging in epidemiological studies. Is it "cause"? Is it "effect"? For example, let us consider scarlet fever. Cases were diagnosed, and these had the typical rash, which was the "result." The "cause," however, was streptococcus, Lansing group A, Griffiths type 4. Moreover, the rash was due to the erythrogenic toxin to which the patient then developed antibodies, so that on the next encounter no rash would be present and thus "scarlet fever" would not be reported. Thus the question is, was the reporting serving a useful purpose or was it occupying medical minds with the least important evidence of infection?

Is illness "epidemic," or is it "endemic"? If epidemic—is it national or international? Again, is it "cause" or "effect" we are recording? If only effect, it may be only one of many and hence may risk obscuring the prime issue. If an organism is endemic, as the word implies, it is a "disease in localities," but then the question is, to what area and also why? This may raise many queries as to source, but in this limited treatise it is proposed to look at "territory." Is it endemic in the area in a general way or is it endemic in families?

My analysis of viral cases in Group 2, shows a 20 percent recurrence rate of viral illness in certain individuals over the years. Obviously, this could not be true of the general populace or the virus would be rife. Also, there is a 10 percent rate of occurrence in a related family member. Again, a 10 percent rate is too high to apply to the general populace.

This is mere observation—what construction do we place on the observation? Also, if we only reported effects, then the figures would be different, for one would have maybe meningitis and another myocarditis, yet both of the same etiology. Thus it seems reasonable to review what we are recording and why. In this connection ME is said by some to be predominantly seen in females. But this is also said of other syndromes, such as myasthenia gravis. Is this true? Looking at the recorded cases in this series, the fact is that if one took CNS cases in total, then ninety-four cases are male. However, the female CNS cases recorded number 225. Among these cases, there are sixty-two male ME cases and 139 female, which is 66 percent male and 62 percent female.

In this series two myasthenia gravis patients were males and two female. One of these females later had a baby, which was affected for the first few months of life and then appeared normal when I last heard of her progress. Again, the total mortality rate for the CNS cases was 7 percent among females and 11.7 percent among males. For ME cases within the CNS groups, the death rate was 9.6 percent among males and 7.0 percent among females, although another syndrome rather than ME was the actual cause of death. This simply means that ME taken in isolation may appear to be more prevalent in the female, but when viewed "in spectrum," it can be seen in a different light.

This familial incidence of infection with the tendency in some to relapse (20 percent) and others to succumb (10 percent), could well account for what we term the "sporadic" cases of infection. This familial incidence challenges the validity of comparing these cases with so-called controls from the general populace; it sounds good but maybe misses the point altogether. Also, if we confine ourselves to a single "effect" or "syndrome," be it scarlet fever or ME, we are certainly taking a tunnel view that has rather serious "field defects." Death among those with CNS sequelae in this series was not always due to the CNS lesion—in some it was concomitant cardiac disease. Further, in some who had cardiac disease and recovered from it—there was still an ongoing CNS problem, causing more disability than the initial cardiac syndrome did. The only common factor that linked the patients was the "cause," in this study, viral.

Moreover, it has been suggested that the day of the hidden virus illness is with us. This seems to be more sinister than the bacterial challenge, for unlike bacteria the virus can be sequestered and the DNA or RNA passed from cell to cell without again entering the general circulation. The development of antiviral as well as antibacterial agents may progress and may in the short term be useful, but once again for the aforementioned reasons it would seem imperative that we address ourselves to research that would give us more understanding of the normal body defenses, which not only eliminate extracellular organisms but can also deal with cells that harbor agents—e.g., virus—or indeed lyse and remove cells that have been damaged by the passage of virus.

This concept should be looked at more carefully. It can be shown in biopsy specimens, in a given field of cells, that some contain viral RNA but most appear clear. Some researchers have assumed that this means the "clear cells" are unaffected. That this is not necessarily so can be shown by studying the metabolism of the cell. Many years ago, before we had the more sophisticated methods now employed, I took muscle biopsies from a patient and one of our microbiologist colleagues made the remark that the cells showed all the signs of "aging," though he could not be more specific. They were muscle cells from a very young man after a coxsackie B virus (CBV) illness. We are now well acquainted with what we term premalignant cell types. Thus we have enough evidence to warrant the statement that cell damage can ensue, certainly by chemical and also by viral means.

It would appear rational to say that cell damage is due to pathology induced within the cell itself, not necessarily killing the cell but interfering with its specialized functions. My observations in patients strongly suggests that in some this interference is perhaps more sinister. Work on Creutzfeldt-Jakob disease has shown how progressive this virally mediated condition can be. In its established form, any effort to lyse all affected cells would be devastating, as it would leave the patient without much functioning brain—it is better to have some than none, we might say! This argues strongly in favor of early rather than late cell lysis. This would inhibit the replication and passage of the virus, thereby halting the slow virus illness. It almost certainly has an application in the field of carcinoma, for now we should be able to see cancer as a process, commencing with the sick cell syndrome and ending in the development of undifferentiated primordial cell lines, which for certain reasons are not effectively removed by the natural killer (NK) cells of the immune system.

In some cases this is due to "coating." For example, certain cell types are coated with HCG as the normal fertilized ovum would be. This coating hinders the scanning recognition of the immune system. This was postulated many years ago, and research has shown it to be true. HCG may be formed on certain cells that have reverted to embryonic form, and yet on others a different lipoprotein coating may be found. However, other reasons emerge whereby the normal "marker" that would be exhibited on the cell membrane and that would make it an NK cell target is either not there or is obscured.

Robert Oldham (1984) of the University of British Columbia in a survey on immunorestoration has made some very fine points. He shows what I have already alluded to and quite frankly tells us that the age of molecular medicine has now begun. Broadly, we may be speaking of lymphokines or cytokines, but laboratory workers are isolating and purifying coded gene products that can correct a varying number of immune deficiency states. These cover areas from congenital to acquired deficiency states that result in inflammatory, autoimmune, and also neoplastic disorders.

Toniolo and colleagues (1984) have done work on both viruses and immunity to show the interrelating effects of both. They point out, however, that studies on the immunological effects of coxsackie viruses are lacking. They show that immunodeficiency is a primary consequence of CBV infection in adult mice and, as stated earlier, this is valid as mice can be conditioned in precisely the same way as humans. These researchers show that CBV types 3, 4, and 6 reduce antibody response to polio virus and heterologous red blood cells (RBCs). CBV also suppresses the generation of cell-mediated responses. In addition, immune responses that depend on T and B cell function are reduced by 50 percent in early infection. Here the evidence is that CBV 3-induced immunodeficiency is due to the malfunction of splenic macrophages.

If normal macrophages become infected, then the plasma cell response to heterologous RBCs is strongly reduced. However, if spleen cells are taken from infected mice and their endogenous macrophages are exchanged for normal adherent cells, the resultant response is normalized. The antigen-presenting cells are altered. Also, CBV 3 appears to activate nonspecific T-suppressor cells. This is another way in which the elimination of infected cells is prevented. It has been shown in experimental work that the thymus, spleen, and lymph nodes decrease in size in the infected host. In mice, spleen weight declined by two-thirds in ten days and the spleen became fibrotic, though the virus itself was not demonstrated. Researchers state that this could be immunopathological in nature or could operate by some other mechanism triggered by CBV 3. My own observation based on other work tends to confirm the theory that the passage of a virus can leave a trail of damage.

Friedman and colleagues (1984) showed and concluded that "the number and function of macrophages both secretory and regulatory can be affected—suppressed maybe at the early stage and changed in function at a later stage to the host detriment e.g., myocarditis, cardiomyopathy, RA [rheumatoid arthritis], etc." It may be noteworthy that RA is a comparatively modern affliction and was not heard of a couple of centuries ago.

Friedman summed up by saying,

> Viruses, which are obligate intracellular parasites, are not only cytolytic for target cells, but also may affect many physio-pharmacologic and immunologic parameters of the host. In particular viruses may influence humoral or cellular immune defenses that develop as protective mechanisms against microbial infection. . . . The type as well as the strain of a virus, the genetic and phenotypic character of the host are all important determinants. Specific receptors on varying cell populations are important for initiating viral replication.

In this connection Professor James Mowbray, Emeritus Professor of Immunopathology at the Imperial College School of Medicine at St. Mary's, London, pointed out at an NRG meeting that even if RNA was discovered in a muscle sample and found to be entero B virus eBv, we would have to be careful as the receptors for eBv could have been on the lymphocytes and maybe when the probe detected the eBv it was actually on lymphocytes in the muscle biopsy and not in the muscle fiber. Some may not agree, but at least it raises the point that we need to be careful in our extrapolation of what we find in an experimental situation—it is the patient that matters. Other factors, however, as divergent as the temperature of the host, the pH of body fluids, and the *virulence de passage* of the virus, serve an important role in delineating the host-parasite relationship in viral infections.

Friedman (1984) went on to show that the humoral mediators, that is lymphokines, monokines, and cytokines, including interferons and interleukins, all have important and not subsidiary roles. He gives a table of the viruses studied and their major effects on the immune system. This fits in perfectly with my own observations, and also it is apparent that this is a changing scene over the years in any one individual and not purely a fixed, inherited state. Thus, he showed that the immunological impairment was due to a functional alteration of the immunocompetent cells. This again fits in with my view that the function of the cell can be changed by virus passage altogether apart from the actual killing of the cell. He states, "the structural integrity of lymphoid tissue does not prevent immunocompetent cells from exhibiting profound manifestations of functional deficiency." For instance, B lymphocyte numbers and function can be markedly altered by viruses, either in vivo or in vitro, in a positive or negative manner. T, B, NK, helper, and suppressor cells can all be affected in this way. Cell surface changes may reduce the ability of cells to interact with endothelial cells or to migrate to appropriate organs. Again, we must differentiate between intracellular pathology that affects cell "life" and membrane pathology that can affect its physiological function in the body. Such changes may be transient or much more permanent. Friedman also showed that the production of interferon by virus-infected cells may have immune regulatory effects. He showed that oncogenesis can occur and that adenovirus types 7 to 11 are oncogenic in hamsters. The messenger RNA of these tumors is virus specific. However, the NK cells in the lysis of tumor cells are "programmed by certain T lymphocytes and adenovirus type 2 is susceptible to a specific T antigen."

Ibelgaufts, with sensitive in situ hybridization methods, analyzed thirty-two human tumors, mainly ectoderm—adenovirus was shown in 62 percent of those tested.

To return to my own observations, over the years it has been difficult to reach a diagnostic conclusion because in many cases atherosclerosis, by virtue of the dicta, was considered to be an etiologic factor in its own right.

During the 1960s, I saw a number of cases that included viral encephalitis, peripheral myositis, myocarditis, Bornholm disease, and also several neonatal CNS abnormalities including brain and spina bifida cases as well as cardiomyopathies. As I stated in a lecture at the time, "it seemed too coincidental and raised the question of the patients having been affected by a prevailing epidemic." During this period I was actively pursuing the poliomyelitis immunization program. This was to be followed by the rubella immunization program, during which cases of encephalitis occurred. Also, during one outbreak of measles some patients also developed encephalitis. It seemed that a changing pattern of viral illness was emerging, and therefore the cases were carefully documented and the ECGs and viral studies were kept.

Other complications arising as sequelae in this series have included the following:

- Peripheral muscle weakness lasting longer than two months occurred in 18 percent of males and 5 percent of females.
- Muscle wasting occurred in 50 percent of these but recovered fairly well later.
- Albuminuria occurred in 32 percent of cases, but was transient.
- Glomerulitis occurred in three, and one case was eventually fatal. One persisted for some months and recovered, but another case appears to be chronic though still surviving.
- Pneumonic: This group includes eight adults with X rays suggesting viral pneumonia; one had some pleural effusion. One resembled miliary TB and is referred to elsewhere. Two babies were affected as described.
- Without any other adenopathy, 4 percent of males had orchitis, and also 6 percent of females had iliac fossa pain suggestive of oophoritis.
- Arteritis developed in four females; two had temporal and two cranial arteritis.

Later, routine study of antibodies became possible, and in the following decade collaboration with a colleague in virology in Scotland resulted in enzyme-linked immunosorbent assay (ELISA) testing becoming a routine procedure for me. Stool cultures were undertaken and proved positive for enteroviruses in about 25 percent of cases, but it also became evident that a time factor was involved, and cultures failed to isolate the organism very soon after the initial infective period. This did not mean that the virus was eliminated, however. IgM and IgG tests were undertaken as well as looking at complement status. These tests did show positive results that suggested the ongoing nature of viral infection and these studies showed that enteroviruses were by far the most common pathological agents. Furthermore, it transpired that the incidence in my locality was similar to that noted in certain Scottish outbreaks (Bell et al., 1988).

However, sera were being sent to Professor Mowbray for the varying complement tests and so on, and a very astute helper in his laboratory decided to mark the house location of cases on a detailed map of this area. It became apparent that most cases occurred in clusters and chiefly on housing estates. The area covered by our general practice includes a number of such estates, chiefly as follows: two estates at Greenside, four at Crawcrook, six at Ryton, four at Blaydon, and four large estates at Winlaton. Only on a rare occasion was a case found in homes or terraces that bordered the main roads. A conjecture that still holds good today was that the common factor was the water supply. The houses on main roads used a supply that was constantly running, while the supply to the estates was more static. The small housing estates had an "end-arterial" water supply. During the night little water would be drawn. The local reservoir water was sampled one year, and it was reported that at the season of bird migration or emigration a 600 percent increase in enterovirus had been found.

Moreover, it was known that enterovirus could be recovered from the cloacae of birds. This seemed too coincidental to be ignored. Hence it seemed, and still appears likely, that birds are one route of spreading infection via the water supply.

It became obvious that varying systems and syndromes were occurring that could not be seen in isolation; moreover, some of these were occurring in family clusters. Other family members in succeeding years became ill. In the hospital setting these would be treated on an individual basis, but in true family medicine it became obvious that there was a distinct family connection both in time and also in the type of illness. This led to serious questioning of previously held concepts. The concept of persistent virus infection became obvious, either a latent infection without obvious harm to the host, or perhaps in some a more subtle illness that hitherto had not been considered as having a viral etiology. Examples range from juvenile diabetes to adult schizophrenia. The cardiomyopathies were more obvious, but again persistent virus infection seemed to be the likely cause, as shown in the case referred to earlier. Consequently, a simple protocol was developed to list these cases. It comprised five groups, which are described in Chapter 1. Later, when the computer came into its own, all this work was computerized except Groups 1 and 2. Those groups are in limbo, but studying ongoing sequential illness necessitated in-depth study of Groups 3, 4, and 5.

Table A and Figure A show not only the numbers of patients by group involved in the study but also the years in which epidemic rises occurred. It is of considerable interest that these rises happened at the same time as those demonstrated independently by Dr. Byron Hyde in Canada and Dr. Betty Dowsett in the south of England.

A further helpful step was the introduction of the VP1 test as developed by Professor Mowbray. It detects viral protein common to the enteroviruses, and it is helpful to relate this to the antibody studies still being performed. However, manual records of serial titers done over the years in certain patients are still required and can be referred to when the need arises.

It has to be remarked that the names of patients often can be confusing in the long computer list and their significance may be missed. This is because of name changes, as in marriage. Numerous cases have occurred where, due to different names, certain illnesses that were familial have not been associated. Obviously, this would be more confusing still in the hospital situation. This occurred in the histories of three sisters who were all ill and in fact died, two due to postviral cardiomyopathy. It was only at the time of death that other members of the family were recognized and the true natural link was established, as their marital names on the computer obviously differed. If this difference could cause an etiologic link to be overlooked by the family doctor, how much more likely would it be in an institutional setting? This problem will be referred to later in Chapter 4. Time intervals of illness, up to years, may also occur and may obscure an etiologic link, which can be very testing to the family doctor and, again, almost impossible in the hospital situation.

TABLE A. Yearly Number of Patients by Outcome Group

Group 1 - New viral illness
Group 2 - Recurrent viral illness
Groups 3&4 - Subsequent ongoing organ pathology
Group 5 - Died

YEAR	GROUP 1	GROUP 2	GROUPS 3&4	GROUP 5	
1954	9	0	1	1	
1955	8	0	1	0	
1956	11	0	2	1	
1957	15	0	1	1	
1958	29	0	1	1	
1959	35	0	8	4	
1960	39	0	2	1	
1961	31	0	0	0	
1962	34	0	2	2	
1963	46	0	4	3	
1964	58	0	6	2	
1965	56	1	2	1	
1966	68	1	5	2	
1967	59	0	1	0	
1968	82	0	5	2	
1969	78	2	6	2	
1970	71	0	9	1	
1971	69	1	3	1	
1972	59	0	10	4	
1973	86	0	9	6	
1974	31	0	13	3	
1975	43	3	10	5	
1976	47	2	10	3	
1977	59	1	15	4	
1978	72	19	42	10	◀ IgG injections
1979	94	18	51	9	commenced
1980	90	18	29	3	
1981	120	24	24	6	
1982	86	16	21	2	
1983	82	13	30	2	
1984	91	17	31	2	
1985	192	14	24	1	
1986	354	69	74	5	
1987	361	97	91	5	
1988	395	97	89	2	
1989	231	107	77	4	
1990	163	81	74	2	
1991	94	54	47	0	
1992	102	46	64	0	

TOTALS	GROUP 1	GROUP 2	GROUPS 3&4	GROUP 5	Decade totals	% Deaths to Groups 3&4
1st decade	257	0	22	14	293	38.89
2nd decade	686	5	56	21	768	27.27
3rd decade	724	114	245	47	1130	16.10
4th decade	1983	582	571	21	3157	3.55
Total	3650	701	894	103	5348	10.33

FIGURE A. Graphic Representation of Yearly Number of Patients by Outcome Group

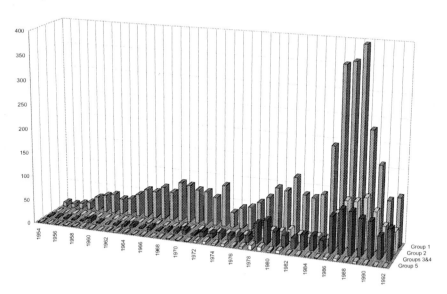

Further challenges to current accepted thought have been brought to light due to this work, including the question of the ability of viruses to reproduce or mutate themselves. This question will be dealt with later in Chapter 1. The concept that only the viral DNA or RNA is harmful might also be challenged, as the prion theory is explored. This type of protein may prove to be derived from sources such as the viral capsid. It might also give Professor Mowbray's work with VP1 as a viral protein more significance and raise the question of VP1's use as a vaccine as well as a marker of persistent viral infection.

Articles published over the past decades are still relevant, and I quote from several in the following sections.

Gerzen, Sweden, BHJ (1972)

The authors showed that myocarditis is not as uncommon as was thought and also quote Levandra-Lindren, who found a high frequency of persisting symptoms, ECG changes, and cardiac enlargement an average of seven years after the initial myocarditis. However, they included nutritional, metabolic, and collagen disease victims in the study. Gerzen did a study, therefore, and their ECG criteria were as follows: transitory repolarization changes defined as repolarization T wave inversion of more than 0.2 millivolts (mV) in at least two leads where the T wave is normally positive. This repeated at least three times. They entered thirty-two male and thirteen female cases. Their patients commonly had precordial pain and a feeling of oppression with tachycardia and dyspnea, and one had acute heart failure. Eleven had a pericordial friction rub (PFR). It was of interest that only three of twenty-six had raised cardiac enzymes. They also showed that the T wave changes were isolated to chest leads 1 to 3. Average convalescence was six weeks, and only three had ECG changes after a year, which were ventricular ectopic (VE) and localized repolarization T wave changes. The authors also showed that orthostatic changes occurred and accentuated the ECG changes by simply moving the patient from the supine to the standing position. They emphasize moving the patient as I have done, and that T wave abnormalities were reproduced most frequently by this orthostatic test. They also state that the stringent ECG changes insisted on probably eliminated a large number of cases with more moderate myocarditis as well as those admitted to the medical ward in acute failure or those in whom sudden death occurred. (Also, my own series would show that pericarditis alone would probably be missed.) However, they also showed that it was not possible in 50 percent of cases to establish the etiology, and they quote evidence to show that viral infection, notably coxsackie B, predominated. Finally, they showed that in the active stage exercise was harmful and recurrences can and do occur. Since then Reyers and Lerner (1988) have shown that making mice swim after infection drastically increases the myocarditis and the chances of a fatal outcome.

Elias Bengttson et al. (1966), Contagious Diseases Hospital, Stockholm

Bengttson and colleagues (1966), showed (again, as we have done) that the ECG changes are not stationary but changed from lead to lead during the acute illness. They were also interested in the myocarditis associated with streptococcal and other conditions. It is interesting that in conclusion they state, "rheumatic and scarlet fever have become infrequent whereas aseptic meningitis has become increasingly common in recent years." They also stated, "The majority of abnormalities found in this presumed viral group also had an incidence of reduced working capacity and enlarged heart volume, at least as great as in the rheumatic group." They conclude that this conflicts with the assumption that viral myocarditis has an invariably good prognosis. Their follow-up after five years showed 20 percent with subjective symptoms and abnormal ECGs and 40 percent with a low working capacity.

G. E. Burch et al. (1967), Department of Medicine, Tulane University

The authors showed that viral antigen can be demonstrated in valves, mural endocardium, and epicardium—using immunofluorescent technique. They showed that the presence of viral antigen is more common than indicated by current literature and is often overlooked. They did their survey in routine autopsy materials, and hearts were randomly selected from fifty-five autopsies of individuals varying in age from stillborn to thirty years. No less than seventeen of these hearts were shown to have a positive result for coxsackie B viral antigen. Three of the hearts also showed an associated mitral valvulitis. Of these seventeen cases, thirteen who had a positive test result showed no significant pathological changes. The authors showed that the lesions were focal and scattered, widely separated, and could easily be overlooked at routine autopsy examination. They conclude by saying, "viral interstitial myocarditis is probably much higher than stated in the literature." They also quote Gold and colleagues in the *New England Journal of Medicine,* who isolated a number of viral agents from infants who succumbed to sudden infant death syndrome. Burch and colleagues (1967) continue by stating, "previous reports indicate that a virus can be isolated from tissues in which there is no histological evidence of inflammation or infection." These techniques readily reveal the presence of viral antigen within the cells. They also suggest that coxsackie B, especially in infants, may be responsible for some forms of cardiac anomalies and that such a syndrome as pulmonary stenosis, which is thought to be congenital, is probably of such an infective origin. Burch suggests that viruses in myocardial cells may remain dormant for long periods of time and may become activated when the body resistance of the host is suddenly reduced by any of a number of factors. This idea, of course, is supported by the behavior of the herpes virus. They also conclude that before acquired valvular disease of the heart (VDH) is accepted as of rheumatic origin, viral etiology should be ruled out.

Rosenberg et al. (1964), **Progress in CVS Disease**

Rosenberg and colleagues (1964) gave a good review and showed that symptoms may be subtle and mimic extracardiac disease. In the adult, signs may include breathlessness, fatigue, and lassitude; in the child simply irritability and poor feeding—until signs of congestive heart failure (CHF) follow. They concluded, as we have done, that no case was an isolated myocarditis but rather that the myocarditis was part of a systemic viral infection.

Adams (1959), **American Journal of Cardiology**

The author reports on eight cases of influenza virus with associated perimyocarditis. The author made the following points:

1. The illness may easily be confused with acute infarction, and the polymorphonuclear leukocytosis is a reflection of the myocarditis just as it is in infarction.
2. The interval between the original infection and the myocarditis is similar to that seen in the onset of acute glomerulonephritis and rheumatic VDH.
3. The author cites twelve fatal cases due to group B Coxsackievirus infection.
4. The so-called postpartum heart disease (i.e., after pregnancy) is almost certainly of viral origin, and they have shown that some are affected during pregnancy. (We have also shown this.)

Sainani et al. (1968), Chicago Medical School

Sainani and colleagues (1968) surveyed twenty-two cases and recovered virus from seven. The other findings included: ECG changes, pleural effusion, pulmonary congestion, and leukocytosis. The average age of patients was forty-nine years. The mean duration of myocarditis was seventy-two months. Alcohol consumption was not found to be a significant factor in these cases. Patients with this myocardial disease did not differ from controls with respect to elevated serum antibody titers of viruses.

Richard Pollen, Georgetown University Medical School, Washington, DC

Finally, Pollen quoted Dalldorf (1948), who isolated coxsackie B from suckling mice and showed that the virus induced a focal myocarditis together with skeletal muscle necrosis and encephalitis and, at times, hepatitis and pancreatitis. The author also showed the advent of pleurodynia, pericarditis, myocarditis, aseptic meningitis, orchitis, and exanthema, as well as deaths in infants, due to coxsackie B infections. They found that other strains could be implicated, including ECHO virus. They concluded by saying that as techniques for the identification of viruses improve, the so-called idiopathic cases will be shown to have viral origin.

This is just a brief résumé of past history but it is perfectly relevant today, albeit maybe not as well recognized as it ought to be. I have seen cases that have slipped through the diagnostic net and were never caught until a fatal outcome occurred, as in the initial cases mentioned in this chapter. Ultimately, the diagnosis was confirmed at autopsy.

The aim, then, in this book is to stimulate research, in relation to the combination of etiologic factors and also host reactions, in individuals, families, and communities.

Chapter 1

Host and Virus Determinants of Organ Pathology

It is obvious that humans are living symbiotically in a world of living organisms. Any organism invading areas outside of its normal habitat becomes pathological. No organism, from humans downward, is pathological providing it remains in its own habitat, and the reverse is true. A good model is *E. coli,* for in the gut they consume some of our food and produce some vitamin B, which is absorbed for the good of the host. In the renal tract, not only is there no "food" for the *E. coli,* but the renal tract is not organized to absorb the bacterial product; thus, so-called infection occurs. In one system *E. coli* is symbiotic and in the other pathological. An unknown number of factors cope with this situation and either render the host "immune" to such invasion, or, if invasion occurs, prevent an ensuing pathological process. Failure of this protective process can occur in many and varied organs and cellular areas. The factors that determine this break in symbiosis or the protection of the species are immeasurably great, and only a few examples can be given here. They are derived from clinical experience and also other scientific works. They serve to explain the diversity of laboratory results, the sequence of varying pathological organic illness in certain patients, and also the observed sequence of family illness.

At the organ level of illness, the work done by Professor Roger Loria (1986b) is very helpful. It could be argued that such illness is not merely at the level of the "organ" in a general sense (e.g., the pancreas), but basically is at the cellular level. This would be relevant because, though we refer to the pancreas in diabetes, it is obvious that in diabetes itself there is widespread pathology of a divergent nature and, as Loria notes, there is a link between diabetes and atherosclerosis.

However, he showed in experiments with mice that there is a genetic role in the development of diabetes in those exposed to coxsackie B4 (CBV4) virus. He used the homozygous diabetic mutant C57Bl/KsJ db/db, which spontaneously develops diabetes, and the heterozygous diabetic mutant C57Bl/KsJ db/+, which remains normal. He showed that in the former (db/db), diabetes could be prevented by restricted diet. In response to CBV4 challenge, however, the order of susceptibility was db/db = (++), db/+ − (+), and those without genetic expression = (−).

More important still was the observation that pancreatic pathology depended upon this genetic mutation. Loria (1986b) showed that in the homozygote db/db, both acinar and islet cell destruction occurred, but in the heterozygote db/+ only acinar cell damage was found. In the normal +/+ mouse only pancreatic inflammation without destruction was found. Thus in the same organ there was a differing response at a cellular level. In his series there was no difference in the CBV titers in other organs of the animals examined. Moreover, at seven days after infection the homozygous db/db strain did not produce any significant level of serological neutralizing antibodies. This proves that the subsequent pathology is not "viral organotrophism" per se, but, as suspected, it is organ or cell susceptibility.

These observations could establish the basis for the concept of organ-specific antibody activity as distinct from more general serological antibody activity. Other examples could be cited to demonstrate the activity of antibodies both in a protective and also in an autoimmune destructive role. The latter is seen, for example, in sympathetic opthalmia. This is considered to be due to antibody formation against pigment released from the iris. Under normal conditions, immuno competent cells never encounter this pigment, but after trauma, when exposed to blood circulation, they do encounter it. One such patient, after a minor graze by a glass particle, developed severe antibody activity in both eyes, and blindness was prevented only by enucleation of the injured eye, in which the sight was perfect.

The series of cases presented in Chapter 5, though limited, does suggest family predisposition to certain conditions following infection: in young people to diabetes, and in the older group to both pancreatitis and ensuing carcinoma, as well as widespread atherosclerosis. It is interesting to postulate that the latter may be a result of lipid abnormality as well. In this regard, it is interesting that, after following up the very young insulin-dependent group for twenty years or more, they do not appear to develop the same severe atherosclerosis, though again this may depend on the genetic mutation of the individual, as shown in Roger Loria's (1986b) mouse model. In this series, however, diabetes and atherosclerosis do appear to be separate entities, albeit when they merge they obviously have a synergistic pathological part to play. It would be helpful to look at a wider group in humans, as Professor J. Banatvala has done, and see if there is a similar genetic determinant for this observed difference in pathological patterns.

John Trentin (1986) showed that the basic pathology of atherosclerosis begins as a nodular, then confluent, overgrowth of smooth muscle cells in the intima of the muscular arteries. It can be observed in this series that if cholesterol is deposited purely because of concentration, then the smaller arteries and capillaries should be affected and obliterated first and foremost. It is obvious that the converse is true, and the larger arteries, such as the aorta and its branches, are the main target. The smooth muscle cells initially invade the intima and the elastic lamina and, as Benditt observed, are atypical in location, size, and preponderance of associated collagen rather than elastin.

Both chemical and viral mutagens were shown to be atherogenic, but again—why? Paterson and colleagues (1950) showed the high incidence of coronary atherosclerosis in avian Marek's disease, which is due to herpesvirus MDV. Since then the atherosclerosis has been established and shown to occur even on a low cholesterol diet. Though high cholesterol aggravates the situation, MDV with low cholesterol is more atherogenic. Moreover, fat itself has a high affinity for viruses, including the coxsackie strains, and in arteries has been shown to convert the muscle cell proliferative lesions to lipoproliferative lesions. Fabricant and colleagues showed that virus-infected smooth muscle cells develop this lipid metabolic imbalance. In addition, cells, during viral invasion, also contain crystals of cholesterol. Benzpyrene and methyl-lcholanthrene, premutagens, contained in cigarettes are transported in blood by low-density lipids, which transport cholesterol as well as viruses.

The pattern would then appear to be viral or chemical lipid-conveyed insult to muscle cell membrane, resulting in these cells losing their inherent localization facility, which results in the invasion of other cell lines—in this case the intima—which starts off the process we call atheroma. It has been shown that these cells have monoclonal X-chromosome expression, which is also a characteristic of virtually all tumors, benign as well as malignant, and this raises the possibility that they may have etiological factors in common. This explains the observed therapeutic value of choline and ascorbic acid in both atherosclerotic and viral disease shown by the author in work done over four decades. Choline is a ptomaine-hydroxyethyl-trimethyl-ammonium-hydroxide, $HO(CH_2)_2N(CH_3)_3OH$. It is known to prevent the deposition of fat in the liver and has benefited diphtheria patients.

I performed a five-year study involving over 400 patients between 1968 and 1973 and represented the results on a graph. Using serum cholesterol levels as a monitor for lipids, the levels showed a marked rise in some patients after choline was administered, reaching a peak in about two months and, thereafter falling gradually to low levels. Moreover, in cases with soft optic arcus this disappeared, and in one or two cases with severe carotid murmurs, the murmurs also disappeared and the patients are still well years later. The addition of ascorbic acid sulfonates the lipids mobilized by the choline and enables renal secretion. This was shown in work done by Dr. R. A. Mumma (1971). It is evident that there could well be a valid reason for giving this mixture to patients who had ongoing enteroviral disease, and over the years this has resulted in the same slow but steady improvement in many. Given the proven lipotrophism of the enterovirus suggested by Roger Loria's (1986a, b) work, the therapeutic modus operandus is self-evident. This is apart from the other functions of choline as a precursor of acetylcholine, etc.

Fujinami and Oldstone (1986) gave suggestions of the complexity of processes that underlie what we call the "household function of the cell." This is a function of the cell membrane, and it is patent that this may be spoiled by viruses, chemicals, or autoimmune processes without necessarily killing the cell. They point out that viruses are known to be polyclonal B cell activators, which can induce production of antibodies and autoantibodies by directly stimulating B lymphocytes, without T cell mediation. Moreover, CBV is known to persist in lymphocytes. Antibodies may form and bind to a viral receptor on a lymphocyte. They then become a mirror image of the cell surface receptor to which they have bound. This is identical to the viral image.

This anti-idiotypic response results in the formation of antibodies, which can bind to the host cell receptors as well as the virus and initiate an autoimmune reaction—a type of molecular mimicry. Thus, if this autoantibody is then attached to a normal cell, it will activate the complement system and lead to cell lysis, or if it does not, other events may ensue and, as suggested earlier, the cell membrane function may be altered. One example would be an autoantibody binding to an acetylcholine receptor site, which would result in a marked decrease in receptor proteins and could be the cause of myasthenia gravis, as noted in three cases in this series. Other household functions would depend on the organ and type of cell involved, but it is not difficult to extrapolate from this to the thyroid, pancreatic islet cells, or even cells of the sinoatrial node or other cells of the cardiac conducting mechanism, as well as the CNS, all of which could have consequences dependent upon the function of that particular organ. The results obviously would be mediated in differing ways: some would be biochemical or hormonal (e.g., thyroid, pancreas, renal, suprarenal etc.), others by so-called "electrical" stimuli (e.g., cardiac or CNS mechanisms). The latter have been shown in this series by ECG and electroencephalogram (EEG) tracings and the former by biochemical assays.

This is a simplistic overview to try to correlate clinical experience with observed laboratory evidence. Further work demonstrates the fact that many other factors must be taken into account.

Professor David Ben-Nathan and colleagues (1994) showed the effects of the pineal neurohormone melatonin on host susceptibility to infection with a virus. He showed that melatonin induces T-helper cells to release opiod peptides, which counteract the immunosuppressive effects of glucocorticoids. The immune-stimulating effects of melatonin were accomplished by the activation of CD4 T cells, which then released the opiod peptides interleukin-2 and interferons. In the treated group of mice (melatonin plus virus) 61 percent died, but in the untreated group (without melatonin), 94 percent died. In an older group, 44 percent of the treated controls died, and in the untreated group, 100 percent died. His work showed that melatonin had no effects on viral culture in cells but exerted its effect by host resistance to virus rather than any direct effect on the virus. He also showed that melatonin stimulates the release of gamma interferon in both human and mouse lymphocytes. It acts synergistically with other mechanisms and as a free oxygen scavenger.

Further work by Melinda A. Beck and colleagues (1995) showed the effects of selenium deficiency, and this formed the basis of experiments in mice. Selenium is a sulfur-like radical that operates in the glutathione complex, a disruption of which results in activity of free oxygen radicals. The ongoing effects of this deficiency were sinister in that a virulent coxsackie virus in the selenium-deficient host had six point mutations of nucleotides 234, 788, 22271, 2438, 3324, and 7334, thereby becoming pathogenic. When this "mutated" virus was transferred to normal mice, the cardiogenic virulence remained. The authors' previous work demonstrated higher virus titers in the hearts of selenium-deficient mice and decreased antigen-specific T cell responses as compared with selenium-adequate mice. They also suggested that an elevated rate of oxidated damage to the RNA genome might occur as a result of the host selenium deficiency. This obviously raises the question of interhost mutation factors and their relevance in the human population.

The role of inorganic elements, such as organophosphates, has been conclusively shown to be sinister as both a factor and a cofactor in human disease. It is over thirty years since one of my patients sprayed insecticides in a room and, within a week, was generally paretic and dysphonic. A diagnosis of acute multiple sclerosis (MS) was at first suggested but, supported by the opinion of an excellent neurologist of the day, a diagnosis of organophosphate toxicity was accepted. Now, thirty years later, this patient has been recorded on video, and all the features are still evident. The acute toxic effects were no doubt due to phosphorylation and subsequent inhibition of acetycholinesterase, while the subsequent limb and spinal muscle weakness probably has an underlying, consequential, pathophysiological mechanism with delayed polyneuropathy. A report titled "Organophosphate Sheep Dip and Human Health—A Seminar for Farmers, Medical Practitioners and Policy Makers" was publisher following a Royal Society conference held in June 1995, in which Dr. Bernhardt gave outstanding evidence of cardiomyopathy developing after exposure to organophosphates. Also,

Dr. Goran Jamal of the Southern General Hospital, Glasgow, showed the impact of organophosphates on the central nervous system.

More recently, I investigated the case of a patient who had returned from a holiday in Turkey. In the hotel where he stayed they had sprayed the rooms against insects, including mosquitoes. His serum levels of varying pesticides, including DDT, lindane, HCB, and p-dichloro-benzene, were significantly raised. Some pesticides have half-lives of many years within the body, and some are used on carpets and soft furnishings as a pesticide. Since he returned, he has been unwell for many months with general malaise and weakness.

Only the tip of the iceberg is evident in reporting the adverse effects of organophosphates, and this is also true when the vast variety of cellular-mediated host responses are considered. This is seen in the cell-line-specific antibody reaction, which is more selective than organ-specific antibody reaction. Examples of this have been seen in biopsy material from the kidneys, liver, and pancreas. In the kidneys after virus infection, glomerulitis was observed with sparing of the nephron, while in the pancreas, destruction of the eyelet cells was evident with sparing of the exocrine cells. This would argue for specific cell-line protection in each organ and, no doubt, could be extended to the variety of particular cell-line constituents of all other organs.

Basically, the cellular constituents of such organs, such as cadherins, have adhesive properties that cause lateral adhesion and have receptors for polar adhesion. All such adhesive binding is homophilic, resulting in one cell binding to the same type within its own domain. The exception to these rigid, structural, organizational mechanisms is seen in the cells of the circulating system, but even these become activated and are concerned with antigen recognition and adhesion under the influence of the immunoglobulin system. These so-called intercellular adhesion molecules find expression on epithelial and endothelial cells and result in the margination and migration of lymphocytes from blood vessels to tissue during the inflammatory response. Figure 1.1 shows capillary margination and migration of leukocytes into adjacent tissue as part of the inflammatory response.

Such defective cell adhesion is obviously present during the invasive and metastatic phases of cancer. Moreover, as shown elsewhere, they lose their membrane specificity and thus, as undifferentiated cells, attract host protective mechanisms such as choriogonadotrophins, which

FIGURE 1.1. Capillary Margination and Migration of Leukocytes into Adjacent Tissue

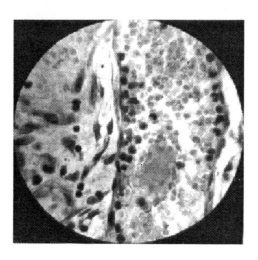

prevent the adhesion of NK cells and allow further tumor growth. Thus the cadherins, integrins, and IgG family of cells participate in a multitude of membrane signals from the membrane afferently to the cell matrix or from the matrix efferently to adjacent cell populations. The development of knowledge with regard to these profound physiological functions will result in the opening of many pathways for the prevention and cure of illness.

GROUP RELATIONS

The patients who had a virus-mediated illness, studied over four decades, number approximately 7,000. As will be seen, five groups have been created during these four decades of research. The group concept became necessary because of the variability of illness, both in severity and subsequent organ pathology. These are not static groups with fixed boundaries, as will be seen when considering the patients and their progress. This in itself demonstrates the variability of illness, both in severity and in time, that may occur in a single patient and also in a family, for a patient may be transferred from one group to another. This observation itself is worthy of thought and has a bearing not only on periods of infection per se, but also on subsequent host activity and environment—chiefly the family environment. Thus the following is an outline of these groups with these considerations.

Group 1

This group was the first to be formed and after four decades comprised approximately 5,000 patients. All the patients in this group had a significant illness of enteroviral etiology but recovered without apparent sequelae within six months. As will be seen later, about 20 percent had a relapse or a recurrence and are listed in Group 2, to which they were transferred.

The acute presentations in Group 1 were varied and included syndromes involving the nervous system, as well as the renal, bowel, pulmonary, glandular, and cardiovascular systems. More general illness, such as a flulike illness with painful myalgia, was very common. This was often the illness we know as Bornholm disease. Other general manifestations were seen in ectodermal tissue such as the skin and eye.

The acute neurological manifestations included viral meningitis and/or encephalitis, an acute cerebellar syndrome in one female only, quite a number of cases of acute labyrinthitis, and also several spinal radiculopathies. These mainly affected the shoulder girdle with gross wasting of scapular muscles, resulting in a "winging" of the scapular.

One of these was videotaped and the tape is interesting to view, the more so as the muscle recovered most of its bulk and now appears normal. More sinister were two cases in the acute stage who developed Guillain-Barré syndrome, which in one case only partially recovered. The cerebellar syndrome could have been mistaken for a vascular incident, while the labyrinthitis cases could have been mistaken for a basilar artery insufficiency.

During the first decade, there was a small outbreak of cases with acute schizophrenia, affecting both males and females. This has been reported by others also. Most of these cases made a full recovery, and the surviving ones still remain well. There was an outbreak here in 1965 of Coxsackievirus group 5, as in Essex also. The latter was reported by Heathfield and colleagues (1967). The Public Health Laboratory Service did show a high incidence of coxsackie B virus group 5, and out of thirty-two cases who were ill and had a positive culture, eleven developed encephalitis and ten meningitis, and two died in the acute stage. However, in this series all of the patients recovered within six months, although in some there was a residual disability, e.g., the case of Guillain-Barré syndrome.

The acute renal cases in Group 1 were all definite but transient episodes of glomerulonephritis, evidenced by repeated positive tests for albuminuria and hematuria. One case was subjected to a needle biopsy that showed a glomerulitis of the kidney. The renal symptoms were superimposed on a febrile flulike illness, but again, most remitted completely within six months. A small number subsequently had to be transferred to Group 3, and two—one male and one female—eventually had to have dialysis, including the case who had the biopsy. The male, a young man, died years later due to a cardiomyopathy that had developed as a concomitant syndrome. He had been transferred to Group 4 and now, of course, appears in Group 5.

The acute bowel symptoms were chiefly seen in those who had a predominantly gastric illness. Several had a subacute phlegmonous gastritis (SAPG), but most had colic and diarrhea. One child had severe SAPG, vomited blood, and had to be transfused, while a young man with a similar presentation had to have a subtotal gastrectomy. He went on to hepatorenal failure and was in intensive care but recovered and was relatively well within six months. With the child, he remained in Group 1. These were all proven cases of enteroviral origin.

The acute pulmonary cases were all cases of viral pneumonitis, and one or two had X rays that mimicked miliary tuberculosis but remitted fairly quickly. Several of these patients developed other organ pathology, either cardiovascular or neurological. When the pulmonary presenting illness remitted, these secondary manifestations became chronic in about 60 percent, and again they had to be transferred to another group. This again illustrates the fluidity of the grouping.

Acute glandular symptoms were rare in the acute stage and chiefly involved the pancreas. One feature marked these cases, which was the tendency to recur and also for subsequent diabetes to develop. Moreover, in one family the father had such an illness and later developed carcinoma of the pancreas and died. His son has had several attacks of viral pancreatitis also but so far has not had the chronic sequelae and is now in Group 2.

The flulike acute myalgias or Bornholm disease were common and occurred in epidemics. These cases have been described nicely by Dr. Wilfred Pickles in his book, *Observations of a Rural Practitioner.* This illness can be absolute agony and require morphine several times daily. Classically, there is a sudden onset of pain, which may mimic an attack of gallstone colic or bowel obstruction or even a myocardial infarction. This passes off usually, only to return in a week or less, and the second attack is often worse than the first. I visited one man about 6 a.m. one morning and videotaped him as he lay in bed, before and after morphine. The videotape is well worth preserving for the education of future doctors. In this series about 20 percent had a third attack about a week later, which was even worse than the first or second. Only a small number had sequelae, but sadly these were severe, and one or two patients in this series succumbed, either to subsequent myocarditis or, in other cases, to gliomas of the brain. Thus some remained in Group 1, but others had to be transferred to Groups 3, 4, or 5.

Finally, ectodermal tissue was not spared, and during the acute stage quite a number of patients developed hand-foot-and-mouth (HFM) disease and/or severe conjunctivitis, and in some an acute iritis. In others, chiefly children, an erythematous patchy rash occurred on the trunk, the thighs, and sometimes on the face. On the tongue and soft palate and tonsils, lesions occurred that closely mimic those seen with eBv infection, but in this group this was excluded serologically as titers for CBV were also shown to be positive. In one family the father and teenage daughter had severe conjunctivitis while the mother had marked HFM disease. Photographs of this family have been retained while all of the other conditions mentioned are on videotape and likewise preserved. They are fascinating to review.

Group 2

It is not proposed to study Group 2, which may be looked upon as a "transitional" group. When the patients followed the pattern of Group 1 and recovered within six months they are retained in Group 2, or, as with Group 1, if other organ involvement occurred they were transferred to Groups 3 or 4.

Groups 3 and 4

Groups 3 and 4 may be considered together. Group 3 comprises cases in which subsequent pathology developed and continued in chronic form in one organ only, while Group 4 comprises those who have multiorgan sequelae. These cases will be more fully described with illustrative histories in the appropriate chapters. However, they do constitute a challenging task, and the early etiology is often quite easily missed. The list of possibilities cited for Group 1 still apply. As Bornholm disease itself is myalgic and usually remits, it can also have further muscle sequelae. This can involve heart muscle, and the number of cases and extent of pathology will be seen in perspective in the section on cardiovascular disease. The renal, CNS, and glandular syndromes all may become chronic. The acute respiratory syndrome of pneumonitis in this series was succeeded by stenosing alveolitis in at least four cases, two males and two females.

The CNS cases were challenging, as in the 1,780 cases listed there have been eighteen gliomas or astrocytomas, which is a very high proportion of cases. These will be referred to in the section on carcinoma in Chapter 8. Other CNS sequelae followed the acute phase, causing patients to be transferred to Groups 3 or 4. These sequelae involved conditions such as a Parkinson-like syndrome, which in a few cases occurred in very young patients; also basal ganglia cell damage with other manifestations occurred in a few. This was described by Peatfield (1987) of Leeds. Two cases in this group developed progressive supranuclear palsy, and they sadly passed through the groups to end in Group 5. These cases are also recorded on videotape.

Glands such as the pancreas and thyroid may also be affected, often by an autoimmune mechanism. Thyroid antibodies occurred eventually in 20 percent of cases, with or without evidence of overt thyroid failure, whereas diabetes ensued in some after initial pancreatitis, and the diabetes was independent of the severity of the pancreatitis. There are well-defined reasons for this, which are discussed in Chapter 5. Other long-term hormonal effects involved the hypothalamic nuclei and their neurohormonal mechanisms, and myasthenia gravis was seen in both male and female cases as an evidence of thymic disturbance. Sleep disturbance, especially the owl syndrome, was found to be common as a late sequel and will be discussed in Chapter 3.

More involved and elusive are the later autoimmune effects, which may affect almost any organ. Three to four decades ago, researchers in the United States advised that viruses should be considered first as initiating agents for mitral stenosis. This applies also to collagen disease elsewhere. Some have progressed to severe rheumatoid arthritis. In this series also, pericarditis has been followed by coronary stenosis free from atheroma, which is discussed in Chapter 2.

An Analysis of Group 5

Group 5 comprises those who died during the time of this study and, as far as can be ascertained, the cause of death was related to the viral illness and its sequelae.

The total number of deaths among 1,783 cases listed is 111, which is 6.36 percent of the whole. Of these 111 cases, seventy were males (63 percent) and forty-one were females (39 percent). The basic pathological cause of death was proven in each case, and four major groups became evident. These have been classified as follows.

Myocardial-Mediated Death

In this group, as will be seen, males preponderate with a total of forty-three cases, which accounted for 61.4 percent of the male deaths. The number for females is sixteen, which is 39 percent. This is in keeping with the figures given in Chapter 2. The ultimate factor varied from dysrythmias to different stages of cardiomyopathy to one case who died after having a cardiac transplant.

Carcinoma-Related Death

Over the years, recurring cases of carcinoma within the central nervous system became obvious, as also were cases of retroperitoneal carcinoma. This observation, coupled with the fact that the usual cases of bowel, breast, and lung carcinoma were absent, has raised a question that may well merit further consideration and research. For these reasons the deaths from carcinoma were self-divided into these two groups. Among males the CNS cases that were either gliomas or astrocytomas numbered nine, which is 12.8 percent of the whole cause of male deaths in the carcinoma group. Among females the corresponding number was four, which is 10 percent of the total. The retroperitoneal cases included eleven males (15.7 percent of the total number of male deaths) and six females (14.6 percent of the female total). In neither group does there appear to be any statistically significant difference in numbers. Only one case of leukemia occurred in a male. This case will be referred to in detail later. The carcinoma cases had earlier been allocated to Group 4 because of multiorgan pathology, but death was ultimately due to carcinoma.

Other Causes of Death

The cases in Group 5 had obviously also been allocated to Group 4, where multiorgan pathology had resulted from viral infection. The pathology included stenosing alveolitis, pancreatitis with or without diabetes, and also some cases of nephropathy. As shown from their inclusion in Group 4, they had other organ pathology, and several died from cardiovascular consequential illness that had been severely exacerbated by some other organ pathology of the same etiological origin. One example was a young man who had hypertension due to previous well-documented viral glomerulitis. He was on dialysis and also had a cardiomyopathy, from which he died, but the total cause of death was multifactorial. Several other patients had severe stenosing alveolitis, which also ended in cardiac failure, with or without a concomitant cardiomyopathy. Thus, in this group, death was due eventually to one organ succumbing to the burden of multiorgan pathology.

From this information, it is obvious that the main single cause of death in this group was either cardiovascular or carcinoma, although other important issues are evident. At the expense of appearing repetitive, I would emphasize that all these cases were "cared for" and the facts are not mere "history." Thus, to survey these cases, a survey of pathology in the cardiovascular cases follows this section.

Summary

- Group 1 contains those who have an acute illness, varying in severity, recovering without sequelae within six months.

- Group 2 may be regarded as a transition group who, again, either recovers completely from a recurrent acute viral illness or develops ongoing organ pathology, either due to persistent viral infection, as discussed later, or due to subsequent virus- initiated autoimmune sequelae.
- Groups 3 and 4 contain the cases with ongoing organ pathology.
- Group 5 contains those who succumb in any of the previous stages.

HISTOPATHOLOGY

Viruses are intracellular obligate parasites, and the host self-protective mechanism has to recognize this. The T cell population only recognizes antigen when it is displayed on cell membranes. T cells then recognize antigen *plus* a surface marker. These markers belong to the major histocompatibility group (MHC). The T helper cells, if primed to the viral antigen, then recognize and bind to it plus the MHC molecule and begin producing interferon (IFN). Thus IFN is synthesized by virus-infected cells and is then secreted into extracellular fluid and binds to the adjacent cells. IFNα is the product of lymphocytes while IFNβ is from fibroblasts and all cell types. The IFN acts on cell genes and frees, or derepresses, two. One of them catalyzes or retards factors responsible for protein synthesis, which therefore reduces mRNA translation, and the other is an enzyme, which causes degradation of host and virus mRNA.

The total result is to establish a cordon of cells around the virus-infected area, which means that viral replication is inhibited. This can be shown in mice, for if interferon is inactivated by an antiserum, they die from a small dose of virus. Thus, interferons have at least three roles: (1) to kill virus, (2) to inhibit host cell division, and (3) to modulate activity of NK cells. Thus it might be said that antibody, complement, and polymorph cells deal with extracellular infections, while T cells, macrophages, NK cells, and interferons deal with intracellular infection. This intracellular infection also can be thwarted by antigenic shift or drift. Antigenic shift involves a change or mutation of viral genome, whereas drift is a swapping of genetic material from reservoirs of different viruses. This could explain the clinical observation that one infection arouses another dormant one of a different strain.

However, both local (i.e., cell) antibodies and systemic (i.e., serum) antibodies function to prevent the spread of virus as it is shed from a cell that it has killed. IgG is the most prevalent antibody of the immunoglobulin system and is a potent opsonizing agent. The complement system of serum proteins is activated initially by IgM and later, more persistently, by IgG. This system opsonizes target cells for phagocytes when it is bound to the IgM or IgG that activated it. This is the classical pathway.

Interleukins (IL) regulate humeral and cellular responses. They are produced by lymphocytes, T cells, and other cell types. IL-1 is produced by both endothelial and epithelial cells and also hemopoietic cells, especially macrophages. IL-1 enhances the immune system by stimulation of T and B cell proliferation, as well as the stimulation of prostaglandins and cytokines such as IL-2, which is excreted by the T cells activated by IL-1. In turn, IL-2 induces T cell toxicity and NK cell activity. Varying changes have been noted to occur in ME cases, suggesting T-cell dysfunction. Hamblin (1983) showed increased spontaneous, T cell suppressor activity and also T cell suppression of in vitro IgG synthesis by normal B cells.

Also, Caligiuri (1987) found that 73 percent of ME cases had a decrease in the number of NK cells, and the T3 negative subset was reduced in 50 percent. Buchwald and colleagues found that stimulation with interleukin-2 resulted in no improvement in cytolytic activity in many patients. They state that the abnormalities of natural killer phenotype and function are interesting, because of the role they play in containing viral infections. Klimas also studied thirty ME cases and found multiple abnormalities of cellular immunity, including decrease in NK cell activity and gamma interferon production. It would appear that there is adequate evidence of deranged immunological activity, and while the pros and cons of IgG therapy are being discussed, this evidence, along with the improvement noted by recipients, would appear to not only validate the treatment but give the reason for its effectiveness. Further work could be done to show the effect on the varying parameters of the immune dysfunctions in these patients after IgG, and thus there would be a more objective measurement of progress.

VIRUS REPLICATION FACTORS

Macrophages nonspecifically take up and kill viruses. This may fail and a virus gain cell entry, and, depending on pathogenicity, it may kill the cell as in lymphocytic choriomeningitis (LCM), Aleutian mink disease, and equine infectious anemia viruses; or without killing the cell, persistent infection may occur.

Surface Antigens

Minor changes or shifts can occur where minor receptor point mutation occurs—this is a minor change in receptor configuration. A major change involves an exchange of genetic material with other viruses. This almost certainly accounts for the observation that during infection with a certain virus, or during a viral epidemic, or during immunization programs, an illness ensues that is not due to the current virus per se, but could be due to a latent virus exchange of genetic material with the new invader. Similarly, an epidemic itself can be due to this drift of genetic material from another virus, causing the so-called mutation of a hitherto noninfectious strain to become pathogenic.

Antibody Activity

Antibody activity may be defined in terms such as the following:

1. *Stereochemical inhibition*—The antibody that coats the cells prevents penetration.
2. *Antibodies to the fusion antigen*—Hinders cell-to-cell spread.
3. *Complement activity*—Augments aggregation and phagocytosis.
4. *Route*—In some cases (e.g., enteroviruses), spreads through bloodstream to target organs, exposing the virus to serological antibodies. This allows the secondary immune response to protect the target organs. In others (e.g., common cold and influenza) the portal of entry is the target organ, and interferon activity is important, but I have shown that surface-acting antibodies work very rapidly and do occur on infected target organs (e.g., the cervix). This involves IgA.

5. *Cell-mediated immunity*—Antibodies can kill virus that is released from killed host cells, but viruses which bud on membranes and spread from cell to cell are not affected by this
means. Examples include oncogenic RNA virus, e.g., murine
leukemogenic, Orthomyxoviridae (flu), *Paramyxovirus* (measles),
togavirus, rhabdovirus (rabies), Arenavirus, (LCM), adenovirus,
herpes (simplex, zoster, CM, Epstein Barr, Marek's) varicella
pox, Papovaviridae, and rubella.

Sensitized T cells are cytotoxic to infected cells and are alerted by
antigens on affected cells. They attack early, as soon as viral antigen
appears, and seem to deprive the virus of host cells. They act synergistically with serum antibodies. Killed virus will induce serum antibodies but not T cell activity, obviously. To me it would appear that while
this is very good it does mean that if a virus gains cell access, this type
of immunity is no longer effective. However, we then resort to:

6. *Lymphokines*—Or the interferons that prevent cell-to-cell spread,
possibly by preventing decoating of the virus capsid (it is a response to non-nucleic acid components).

Thus, as seen in the first section, the host response is complex, and,
as summarized here, the interaction between host and virus to prevent
disease is also complex. Our survival owes immeasurably more to the
immune system than it ever will to "medicine," and perhaps we have
more lessons to learn by research into this symbiotic system.

Chapter 2
Cardiovascular Consequences of Viral Infections

HISTORICAL BACKGROUND

Christian, in an article in 1951, showed that as long ago as 1854 idiopathic pericarditis was an acknowledged disease. Benign pericarditis and also idiopathic myocarditis, as well as chronic cardiomyopathy, were also recognized as fairly common entities long before a possible viral origin was suspected. Indeed, I have a death certificate from the 1920s that gives myocarditis as the cause of death. Mitral lesions likewise were constantly attributed to a streptococcus-induced rheumatic infection for decades after streptococcus-induced rheumatic fever had almost disappeared. It is only since the late 1950s that the viral etiology has been recognized as important and a huge relevant literature has appeared. Many have observed that before streptococcus hemolyticus is considered to be the etiological agent, the viral origin should be considered and sought for. In the family studies reported in this chapter where myocarditis was the designated cause of death given on the death certificate, and the viral etiology had been established, it could be shown that in some cases other family members had succumbed to virus-induced cardiovascular pathology.

Woodruff (1980) published a review in which he showed that many illnesses were incriminated in these processes, including infectious mononucleosis, measles, smallpox, poliomyelitis, influenza, and more common than these were the Coxsackieviruses. It was shown at the time of the polio epidemics that 20 percent of polio cases developed myocarditis, and a significant number died of it. Professor Roger Loria (1986a) has shown that after any significant illness due to coxsackie infection, 5 percent of the cases developed a cardiac lesion. During the severe influenza epidemics, a similar number succumbed in a similar manner. This occurred after World War I and, in a smaller number of outbreaks, has done so sporadically since then. However, the enteroviruses remain one of the most common causes of virus-mediated pathology, and this chapter deals with the cardiovascular consequences of this infection.

PRESENT SERIES

In the series to be presented here, a similar percentage of cardiac lesions occurred after enteroviral infections. These infections include the enteric cytopathic human orphan (ECHO) and coxsackie viral strains, both B and A, though until the 1970s titers for the latter were not available, and we had to depend on stool cultures. No doubt the numbers would have been greater had we been able to do cultures in all cases. There is speculation as to whether other viruses such as the adeno and retroviruses as well as the herpes group can also be involved. Viruses, especially the enteroviruses, have been isolated from myocardial tissue during catheterization or at transplantation. This series includes both congenital and acquired disease after viral infection.

In the congenital cases we have detected congenital anomalies resulting from infection in the first trimester of pregnancy, which caused agenesis or malformation in one or more organs, whereas infection in the second and third trimesters resulted in injury to the fully developed organ. Examples of first-trimester infection include cardiac defects such as septal lesions, when an audible systolic murmur was present at birth, and brain defects such as agenesis of the septum pellucidum when quite early the baby was seen to be blind. In late-trimester infections damage was also seen in cardiac and brain tissue. In the cardiac cases, several neonates developed a marked systolic heart murmur within a week or two of birth and died within a year. At postmortem examination endocardial fibroelastosis was obvious. In other neonates, septal abnormalities occurred. Some of these were amenable to correction and open heart surgery was performed. The earliest of these was a tetralogy of Fallot, which was successfully dealt with in sequential stages, and the patient is now a married man. In the brain, late-trimester infection resulted in destructive lesions, which will be discussed in Chapter 3.

In acquired disease, chiefly in adults, various patterns of cardiac disease as well as pathology in other organs occurred, varying from mild to lethal. Thus, pericarditis alone was seen in eighty-two female patients and manifested by a pericardial friction rub without ECG changes. There were only two deaths in this group; one was due to a subsequent brain tumor and the other to a retroperitoneal carcinoma following a subsequent virus-mediated pancreatitis. Male patients numbered seventy-five, and only one death occurred, in this case also due to carcinoma of the pancreas years later. He had had viral pancreatitis at the time of his pericarditis. Thus, pericarditis may be relatively benign though painful at times, varying with body position and often worse when the patient is lying on the left side, though it may occur as high as the manubrium and could raise doubt as to other pathology. It might be construed as a mediastinitis analogous to pleurisy; and, as the lung is spared in pleurisy, so the myocardium can be spared in mediastinitis or pericarditis.

In this series a definitive friction rub, with significant chest pain but without ECG changes, was considered to indicate pericarditis. Not all cardiologists would agree, and it may be hard to prove or disprove, but the fact that a change of position will aggravate the pain and exacerbate a PFR seems to warrant the assumption. The term "perimyocarditis" was used for the next stage, where the myocardium was seen to be involved, as shown by ECG changes.

In the pericarditis cases the following should be noted. Almost any virus can be the causative agent, with coxsackie B virus being by far the most common in this series. The signs of pericarditis are interesting, for the visceral pericardium is insensitive to pain while the lower pericardium is supplied by fibers from the intercostal and phrenic nerves. The pain due to pericarditis is usually stabbing in character and is made worse by breathing, coughing, body movements, swallowing, and, typically, by lying on the left side in bed. It may radiate to the front of the chest and, among the cases described here, many have had pain in the left arm, but it has been noted that whereas referred cardiac anginal pain is in the ulnar border of the arm, pericardial pain is in the outer or radial border. I find this sign of considerable significance. Because of this, I often use the term "mediastinitis," as it relates to the parietal pericardium in which the nerve fibers are located, and hence the outer border of the arm is the site of the referred pain. We have found that ECG changes show a mild upward deviation of ST segments in the limb leads and also leads V2 to V6. Case F13, detailed in the case report in the perimyocarditis section, illustrates these points.

Sixty-four male and seventy female cases were recorded in this series. The subsequent death rate was higher than that seen in the pericarditis cases, but in only two cases was death caused by cardiac failure. One was in a man in his late forties. The other was in a young man in his thirties who had had quite severe perimyocarditis and also nephritis, for which he eventually required dialysis. He was found dead in his bed, and at postmortem examination he had gross atherosclerosis of his coronary arteries. Since coronary arteries lie so close to the actual myocardium, their involvement in perimyocarditis is not surprising.

No doubt atheroma is the most frequent cause of coronary artery disease (and this can be shown to be multifactorial), but a number of cases with well-documented perimyocarditis later developed angina and had coronary artery surgery with grafting and on histology "coronary artery stenosis without atheroma" was reported. One such patient had a six-vessel coronary graft, and each section was reported as showing stenosis free from atheroma. This may be considered to be a process similar to mitral stenosis, in which collagen is the tissue affected. This caused a similar constrictive lesion. In the myocardium, varying degrees of inflammation or fibrosis may occur. This can be fulminating, manifesting as congestive cardiomyopathy and requiring transplant, or chronic, resulting in either a hypertrophic or a dilated cardiomyopathy.

In this series, myocarditis occurred in forty males and thirty-six females. As stated earlier, the death rate was different in this group, and sixteen males but only five females succumbed, representing for the males a 40 percent and for the females an 13.8 percent death rate. Fuster in 1981 described this syndrome clinically as a "diffuse, global decrease in amplitude of contraction," and it is interesting that this mirrors the process seen in peripheral muscle due to virus-mediated myositis and also in some cases where fatigue, softening, and sometimes infarcts in muscle also occur. Moreover, the prognosis was paralleled by the degree of dilation, as expected.

In other cases in this series, endocarditis also occurred. In neonates this manifested itself in two cases as endocardial fibroelastosis, which was mentioned earlier (see patient F18 in Chapter 7, and Figure 4.3). Three cases in adults manifested by papillary muscle inflammation and necrosis, leading to valve leaflet prolapse. One such case required valve replacement, and during the open heart operation it was interesting to view the chordae tendineae "loose and flapping" while the papillary muscles were almost nonexistent. Also, the retropropulsion of blood through the mitral valve caused a "gyration" of the heart at each beat; following the insertion of the valve prosthesis this gyration was clearly absent. This patient, who is currently quite well, had also previously suffered an episode of bacterial endocarditis following the previous well-defined coxsackie myocarditis. Some time afterward he developed a mitral systolic murmur, which was considered to be due to the prolapse of one of his mitral leaflets. Later a diastolic murmur became evident, which suggested that both leaflets had prolapsed. This was confirmed at operation.

In another case, at operation the myocardium was seen to be infarcted at the origin of the papillary muscles, and transplant of the muscles into healthy myocardium was successfully achieved. Other anomalies occurred, including one male in his late fifties, many years ago, who, subsequent to his viral myocarditis, had ventricular extrasystoles that occurred with continuous regularity, as seen on the ECG. He was found to have a small fibrotic "node" in the left ventricle, which was maybe acting as a capacitor and discharging with regularity. No doubt this was due to the previous viral myocarditis. At that time he was sent to London, where this nodule was removed, and postoperatively his heart restored a normal rhythm. So far constrictive pericarditis has not been a sequel in this series.

Two heart transplants were performed in this series. One was in a young man, referred to later, and he did well as it was early; the other was in an older man in the stage of dilated cardiomyopathy, and he only survived a few months. It would appear from the postmortem report that he died because of rejection of the transplanted heart.

Epidemiology

The true incidence of viral myocarditis as a cause of sudden death is not known, but Woodruff (1980), Loria (1986a), and this series show that 5 percent of viral infections cause some cardiac involvement. In a study of 40,000 unselected cases coming to autopsy, Smith (1970) reported that of the 417 young and middle-aged victims and 214 children who died suddenly, myocarditis of suspected viral origin accounted for up to 5 percent of the deaths. In another three-year study of ninety Minnesota children who died before reaching seventeen years of age in 1970, 7 percent died from this condition, while a Japanese survey in the same period (1970) of forty-seven sudden deaths in schoolchildren showed that 21 percent had myocarditis. Also, during epidemics of Coxsackievirus, lethal myocarditis occurs in some 50 percent of infected infants (Woodruff, 1980).

In the series reported here the seasonal incidence is evident, in that sporadic cases that are endemic and involve coxsackie groups 2 and 4 are different from those which involve coxsackie groups 1, 3, and 5. The latter occur during the spring and autumn and are epidemic. This has been surveyed over four decades, and it can be shown that these were epidemic infections probably due to contamination by birds congregating at reservoirs during migration and emigration. One year a 600-fold increase in recoverable enterovirus was found in local reservoir water. In that year there was a drought, and the reservoir water was low and hence concentrated, thus raising the concentration of the virus. Also, epidemic mortality has been seen in frogs and other aquatic creatures, as well as land animals such as foxes, and this has been attributed to viruses. Humans, by drinking the water, become infected hosts and may then harbor and mutate the virus, which is then excreted, and further pollution occurs.

Sex

In this series as well as that of Woodruff (1980), as shown in the previous section, males were more likely to die, though females were as susceptible in the acute phase. This sex difference was not apparent in the congenital cases, but the numbers were small. Males in this group did progress to cardiomyopathy more often, which was related to the greater manual labor of males. Cardiomyopathy has been shown in mice infected by Coxsackievirus. The infected mice developed myocarditis, but if placed in water where they were compelled to swim, they then developed a cardiomyopathy irrespective of sex, for both sexes were similarly stressed, unlike the human groups (Reyers and Lerner, 1988).

Cofactors and Adjuvant Syndromes

Alcoholism was excluded as a contributory cause in this series, although it must be stated that these patients are very sensitive to alcohol, which can act as a severe cofactor, especially in cardiac disease. This also applies to cigarette smoking. Professor Loria (1988) in his published work showed the marked effects of cholesterol in coxsackie-infected mice. The virus insult to the vascular endothelium is followed by cholesterol crystal deposition with ongoing pathology, which may be avoided by putting mice on a low-cholesterol diet. It is interesting that Professor Duguid, while in Newcastle, also demonstrated this synergism of pathological cofactors in arterial disease as long ago as the 1940s (personal communication).

As happened in cases who had poliomyelitis, influenza, and the other diseases mentioned, myocarditis can easily be overlooked, as it may be less distressing to the patient than the other manifestations of their current illness. The results in this series did show that some died from just such an unsuspected myocarditis, while in others a known myocarditis resolved but left the patient still feeling ill due to the other systemic effects of the original infection. These effects could vary from polymyositis or Still's disease to diabetes or myalgic encephalomyelitis. It is interesting that a recent paper showing the prevalence of cardiac abnormalities in an ME cohort validates the results observed over the decades here (Lerner).

Histology

In myocarditis, an infiltration of monocytes with myofibril inflammation and some necrosis is seen. These monocytes have been shown to play a critical role in suppressing viral growth. In this group cortisone did not help, but seemed to activate the disease process; it is suggested that this is due to diminishing macrophage activity. Woodruff (1980) noted this effect also and showed that macrophages from the peritoneal cavity of uninfected mice suppressed viral activity in an infected host. However, this occurred in the early stage of infection, and later, when T cell activity occurs, their function may be altered by T cell antibody-dependent, cell-mediated cytotoxicity, resulting in damage to myofibrils. This effect could be seen as the autoimmune result following the acute infection and, again, in our series can be marked, though not consistently, by a rise in erythrocyte sedimentation rate (ESR). If this was high, e.g., 80 mm in one hour (Westergren method), then cortisone might be helpful at this later stage. In my experience, the early use of immunoglobulin may prevent the occurrence of this stage. This could well be due to the activation of the T cell immunity mechanism.

In various papers reports have shown the beneficial effects of immune serum IgG administered at the time of infection and its protective role against lethal disease. This has been my experience over three decades and remains a cornerstone of therapy. In 1980, Woodruff also showed that the adult form of myocarditis was histologically similar to that found in the neonates and could cause inflammation of the atrioventricular septum bundle of His. In the latter, fibrosis has been a late feature and no doubt this, together with inflammation near the sinoatrial (S=A) and atrioventricular (A=V) nodes, can account for some of the ECG changes and the clinical abnormalities in rhythm that have been shown in both the acute and chronic phases.

Electrocardiograms

A varied pattern of change can occur that may be reversible and also recurrent, or later chronic. P wave abnormalities may occur, and P-R interval changes suggesting a Wenckebach type of lesion are sometimes seen. Atrial Ventrical Repolarization (QRST) conduction changes suggesting bundle-branch block have been seen and may remit or be more or less permanent, suggesting pathology to the bundle of His, alluded to earlier. Ventricular ectopic (VE) beats frequently have been seen and may be variable or have a more regular pattern as shown earlier. A peculiar biphasic repolarization T wave that resembles an N may occur. This, I suggest, may be evidence of repolarization commencing, as it should, on the inner myocardium and then being overtaken by activity from the outer myocardium, resulting in the "negative" deflection. A very high T wave may occur as evidence of an unstable and inflamed myocardium.

As mentioned earlier, it has been shown in the chronic stage that a discrete fibrotic area may act similar to the A=V node as a "capacitor" and initiate ectopic VEs in the same way as the A=V node. The excision of one such fibrotic lesion in a male resolved the condition, and no further ectopic beats occurred. In the more acute stage, changes in the repolarization T waves can vary from day to day. On one occasion they may be inverted in chest leads 2 and 3 but be upright in leads 4, 5, and 6 and days later be upright in chest leads 2 and 3 but be inverted in 4 or 5 or 6. This suggests the migratory pattern of inflammation in the myocardium.

The numbers in Table 2.1 represent the cardiac sequelae. From these statistics, it is very obvious that the number of males was higher only in the cardiomyopathy group in this series. This is substantiated by Woodruff (1980), as he also showed this difference in male and female mice in the acute stage. The mortality ratio, however, shows a gross preponderance of males. CVS deaths account for 55.8 percent of the whole series, and, of this total, male deaths account for 70 percent and females for 30 percent. Again, this is entirely in keeping with the figures published by Szentivanyi and colleagues.

Comparative Total Cardiovascular Mortality

Of the 1,783 cases being considered, ninety-five resulted in mortality. They constitute Group 5, 5.3 percent of the total. Of these, fifty-three died of cardiovascular disease, i.e., 55.8 percent of the deaths. This can be subdivided by sex as follows:

Males   37   70 percent of the total
Females   16   30 percent of the total

In the study of mortality some facts emerge that are of interest. The first is the prominent sex difference, with the number of male cases being more than twice that of females. This, as shown, was due to the cardiomyopathy group in the main. The second observation is that, as shown earlier, not all deaths were due to cardiac disease. The other groups are summarized in the following sections.

Pericarditis Group

Males   Seventy-five cases with only one death (1.3 percent), which was due to carcinoma of the pancreas. This also followed a previous viral pancreatitis.

Females   Eighty-two cases with two deaths: in one a glioma of the brain subsequent to the original infection, and in the other a retroperitoneal carcinoma subsequent to a viral pancreatitis that occurred at the same time as the cardiac lesion.

TABLE 2.1. Cardiac Sequelae

	Total CVS Cases	CVS with Another Syndrome (CNS or gland, etc.)	CVS Alone
Males			
Pericarditis	74	28	46
Perimyocarditis	54	35	19
Myocarditis	35	10	25
Cardiomyopathy	19	3	16
Total	182	76	106
Females			
Pericarditis	86	47	39
Perimyocarditis	70	46	24
Myocarditis	36	18	18
Cardiomyopathy	4	3	1
Total	196	114	82
Grand totals			
Males	182	76	106
Females	196	114	82
All	378	190	188

Perimyocarditis Group

Males   Sixty-four cases with ten deaths (15.6 percent). Of these, only three were attributable to cardiac disease. Two cases died from stenosing alveolitis that followed the initial acute viral pneumonitis, and five died from retroperitoneal carcinoma, again following viral pancreatitis.

Females   Seventy cases with no deaths.

Myocarditis Group

Males   Forty cases with sixteen deaths (40 percent). In this series, by contrast, only three deaths were unrelated to cardiac disease and were due to stenosing alveolitis, again following viral pneumonitis.

Females   Thirty-six cases with five deaths (13.8 percent). Only one case was not related to the cardiac disease, this being due to carcinoma of the pancreas following a pancreatitis of the same viral etiology.

Dysrythmia Group

Examples of those who died of dysrythmias include a female who, while cleaning the windows of her car, collapsed and died. Another young man got into his car to go to work and died before he could start the engine. A young man in his twenties was found dead on the pavement on his way to work. A third young man came home and, not feeling well, went to bed in a separate room, as his wife was five months pregnant; unhappily she found him dead the following morning. The fourth case was a man in his fifties who was recovering from a viral myocarditis. He was returning with his wife from a holiday abroad and likewise collapsed and died before he could reach the car awaiting them. All of these cases had proven coxsackie-mediated myocarditis, evidenced by serological titers and serial ECGs.

Heart Surgery Group

Those in the heart surgery group were all male. Two had heart transplants, one in his late teens and the other in his late forties. As seen elsewhere, the former survived and the latter died. Three had operations for valvular prolapse, all of which involved the mitral valves. Three cases were subjected to coronary grafts, one with six vessel grafts; all were reported as having stenosis without atheroma, as discussed earlier.

Unexpected Sudden Deaths

The number of sudden deaths merits detailed consideration. Six of the patients were male and two were female, and all were in the twenty to forty-nine age group. They all succumbed to dysrythmias except one female, who died from a rupture of the left ventricle, resulting in a hemopericardium, and two males who were found dead in their beds. The postmortems both demonstrated pathology identical to the first case mentioned in the Introduction and were considered to be related to previous cardiomyopathies.

ANECDOTAL CASE REPORTS

This section gives details of proven cases, divided into five groups as shown, and then subdivided into male and female patients. Most are from Group 5, the fatal outcome group, as these were mostly proven by autopsy. Only two or three cases have been randomly selected for each group as illustrations. In reading these brief reports, it is well for the reader to consider that these are not just numbers, but rather that they represent many poignant experiences and countless hours spent with patients and families in their suffering.

The cases are grouped under the following headings:

1. *Myocarditis acute*—those recovering or dying within two years of the initial illness
2. *Myocarditis relapsing*—cases who recovered or died during a relapse years later
3. *Cardiomyopathy*—chronic cases developing cardiomyopathy
4. *Myocarditis with other syndromes*—those who developed another viral related illness
5. *Perimyocarditis*

Myocarditis Acute Group

Male Patients

No. 1. M01, DOB 1957. Diagnosed and died 1974. This was a young man in the armed forces who presented with a viral illness and was breathless and had chest discomfort. He was admitted to a hospital under the care of one of my colleagues, and at first it was thought that he had had a myocardial infarction. He developed a low-grade fever, and subsequent serial ECGs (see Figure 2.1) showed the patterns of

FIGURE 2.1. M01's ECG

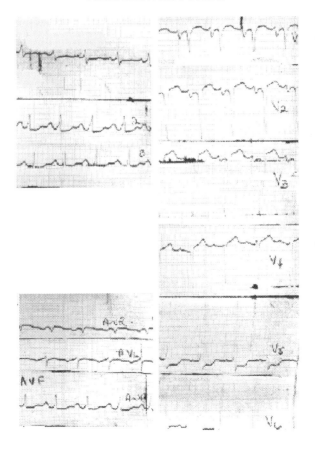

viral myocarditis with abnormal T wave configuration in the chest leads, changing from day to day in location from V2 to V6. This suggested the migratory pattern of inflammation seen so often in myocarditis. His serial titers of coxsackie B group 4 rose to 1/512 with a positive ELISA IgM and IgG. After several months of illness, he died of congestive cardiomyopathy. Had this occurred today he would almost certainly have received a transplant, and his life saved. Postmortem examination demonstrated a pale flabby heart with the typical cellular infiltrate of monocytes.

No. 2. M02, DOB 1946. Diagnosed and died 1981. This was a young family man whom I knew very well, who became ill and exhibited a classical history of viral infection. His titers of coxsackie B group 4 rose to 1/128 and he later had a positive test for IgM. He developed myocarditis, and routine ECG changes were identical to those of case M01. In addition, he had some ventricular ectopic beats, and one or two dysrythmic attacks were recorded. Over the subsequent months he appeared to be remitting, and his ECG improved and appeared stable. He said he felt generally well and returned to work on his own volition. One morning he left home and got into his car to drive to his office. His wife did not hear the engine start but saw his foot protruding from the open car door and thought he was looking into the glove compartment. As he did not move, she went down and found that he had died. A postmortem was performed and demonstrated the myocarditis and found the coronary arteries clear of atheroma. It was thus judged that he had died from a further dysrhythmia.

No. 3. M03, a sixty-two year old man who came from Greece in February 1974. This man presented with palpitations, chest discomfort, photophobia, malaise, and acute breathlessness. On examination he had a supraventricular tachycardia of 120 beats per minute and the peculiar N-shaped T waves seen on leads L3, AVF, and V5 (Figure 2.2a). His blood pressure (BP) was normal as was his blood urea, cholesterol, and other blood chemistry. Because of his acute symptoms, under ECG monitoring, I initially gave him IV practolol, resulting in a stable ECG as shown (see Figure 2.2b). ECHO virus group 4 was isolated from his feces. There was an epidemic of ECHO viral infection that year, of which further examples are described among the female cases. As it was obvious that this was an acute viral myocarditis, he was treated with intramuscular IgG 750 mg weekly and,

FIGURE 2.2a. M03's ECG Before Practolol

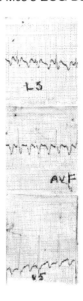

FIGURE 2.2b. M03's ECG After Practolol

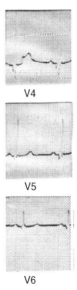

V4

V5

V6

though he had a stormy passage, he made a good recovery, moved away, and came to see me a year later when he was very well, with his ECG remaining normal.

No. 4. M04, DOB 1971. Diagnosed 1987. This young man belongs to a family in which the effects of Coxsackievirus infection have been particularly lethal. His mother had episodes of encephalitis and meningitis, and a baby born during this period died due to endocardial fibroelastosis during its first year. The young man presented with the usual symptoms of dyspnea and chest oppression. Knowing the history of the family, he was very carefully examined and was found to have all the signs and symptoms of viral myocarditis. His blood showed a sixteenfold rise in coxsackie B group 3 titer and a positive ELISA IgM and IgG. Later he had a positive virus protein 1 (VP1), a capsid genome (see Figure 2.3).

FIGURE 2.3. M04's ECG

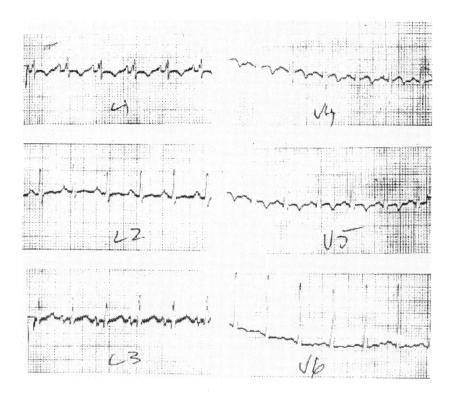

He was referred urgently to a hospital, and a cardiac transplant was performed. Subsequently his cytomegalovirus titers rose to 1/512 and the IgM again was positive. He is maintained on therapy to prevent graft rejection, and so far the outcome has been satisfactory.

Female Patients

No. 1. F01, DOB 1964. Diagnosed and died 1979. This young woman was seen with an illness of the Bornholm disease type with chest and upper abdominal pain. It remitted and recurred four days later. Subsequent tests showed high titers of coxsackie B group 4 of 1/512 and groups 2, 3, and 4 of 1/32. Other members of the family also had high titers of the same coxsackie grouping. This is referred to in 4. Sadly, she was found dead in the garden, and it was erroneously supposed that her horse had kicked her, as its hoofprints surrounded her where she lay on the snow-covered ground. However, no sign of injury was found, and it was apparent that the horse had merely been "concerned" about its owner. Postmortem showed signs of acute myocarditis. No ECGs were performed in this case because myocarditis was not suspected at the time. This again should be a warning to us that initial diagnosis might be misleading and that more serious pathology should be considered.

No. 2. F02, DOB 1952. Diagnosed 1970. Died 1971. This young woman had a typical viral illness in the last term of pregnancy. She also had rising coxsackie B titers as follows: B1 = 16, B2 = 32, B3 = 32, B4 = 512. She had ELISA positive IgM and a positive stool culture. Initially her illness presented as a typical viral pneumonitis, which this later remitted, but labor appeared to have an adverse result in her case. She developed a perimyocarditis, as evidenced by a friction rub and ECG changes. The outcome of labor appeared to be initially satisfactory. However, I later learned that the baby was affected, but the full details are not known as she moved from the area. In the neighboring town she came under the care of a colleague of mine, as she was still suffering from myocarditis. I spoke to him concerning the initial phases of her illness, and he took a great deal of interest in her case. Unhappily, I was later informed by her mother that she had been traveling with her husband in his car when she suddenly slumped forward. He rushed her to the nearby hospital, but on arrival she was found to be dead. The postmortem findings again indicated myocarditis. This case illustrates the difficulties that arise if adequate diagnosis and case notes of the original history are not available, or if they are available, the significance is not at first fully appreciated.

No. 3. F03, DOB 1943. Diagnosed 1973. This female had episodes of chest oppression, feelings of faintness, and pain some weeks following a viral illness. ECHO type 4 virus was isolated from her feces. This was in a year when ECHO virus illness was epidemic. On examination she was discovered to have a pulsus quadrigeminus, the ventricular ectopic beat evidenced by one missed beat in every four on auscultation and confirmed by the ECG shown in Figure 2.4. It was of interest that the date

FIGURE 2.4. F03's ECG

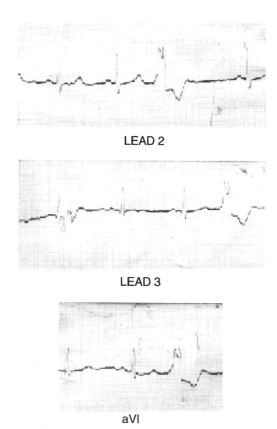

LEAD 2

LEAD 3

aVl

of her last menstrual period suggested that she had conceived, and she subsequently bore a normal baby. It would have been easy to pass over the viral infection in this case as it was acute and she made a good recovery. Her ECGs later became normal and have remained so. This was a very happy outcome different from some others, and thus is worth recording.

No. 4. F04, DOB 1948. Diagnosed 1974. A young woman in the same age group with a pattern of illness and conception identical to F03. It was less than one year later, and she also had a pulsus quadrigeminus as confirmed by ECG (see Figure 2.5). An identical strain of ECHO virus was cultured from feces, as in many other cases during this epidemic. She happily had a normal pregnancy with delivery of a normal baby in February 1975. Subsequently her ECG normalized, and she and the child have happily remained well since then. This, again, is an outcome worth recording.

Myocarditis Relapsing Group

Male Patients

No. 1. M05, DOB 1945. Diagnosed 1971 and died 1976. In the epidemic year 1971, this young man initially presented with a flulike ill-

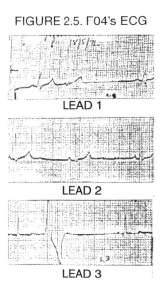

FIGURE 2.5. Г04's ECG

LEAD 1

LEAD 2

LEAD 3

ness and a typical Bornholm disease. His titers of coxsackie B group 4 rose to 1/512, with positive IgM and IgG and a positive feces culture. His ECG also showed migratory T wave changes in the chest leads and ventricular ectopic beats with one or two episodes of dysrythmia. After a somewhat stormy few months he seemed to recover and his ECG normalized. This illness lasted well over two years, but, as he then felt so well, he decided to return to work. This involved traveling, and he appeared to be managing without any recurrence of symptoms for well over a year before he had an attack of palpitations while on a business trip in Scotland. He was admitted to hospital due to palpitations and breathlessness and died. Postmortem examination in the hospital showed a patchy inflammatory myocardium with clear coronary arteries, and a postmortem diagnosis of myocarditis was given on his death certificate.

No. 2. M06, DOB 1951. Diagnosed 1981 and died 1983. This young man had a rather severe attack of Bornholm disease with typical gripping pain in the upper abdominal wall. This remitted, but many months later it was followed by some chest discomfort. Once again the ECGs were classical for an acute myocarditis, but this appeared to resolve fairly rapidly, and he did not have any dysrythmia. Serial titers to coxsackie B group 4 again showed a rise to 1/512, which over subsequent weeks fell to 1/32. He also had IgM and IgG complexes and a positive stool culture. He appeared to recover well and returned to work. Later his wife became pregnant, and I was asked to book her for a home delivery, which was expected in April 1984. However, he apparently felt ill again at Christmastime but did not consult me and went out on New Year's Eve. His wife told me that he returned home and, due to not feeling well, went into another bedroom to "leave her in peace." On going to waken him the following morning, she found him lying dead in his bed. Postmortem examination showed the changes of myocarditis with clear coronary arteries. I delivered the baby in April as arranged, and he was given his father's name as had been agreed upon previously. As the mother had not had any illness I expected all would be normal with the baby, and happily this proved to be correct, which was a great consolation.

No. 3. M07, DOB 1925. Diagnosed 1974. This man was in his forties when he came home from a holiday in Malta and was acutely ill with an attack of Bornholm disease. He had a coxsackie B group 2 titer of 1/32 and group 4 titer of 1/1024. He also had a positive IgM and later IgG and a lowered complement (CH50 = 20). He made a slow recovery, but then had a relapse and developed typical viral myocarditis. Serial ECGs demonstrated a changing pattern of the repolarization T waves in the precordial leads from week to week. This was considered evidence of a migrating inflammatory process. Subsequently, he had some stormy years and was the subject of considerable medical care, during which he had an episode of bacterial endocarditis in 1981. It resolved very satisfactorily on antibiotic therapy, but some years later he had another relapse due to the Coxsackievirus and developed an apical systolic murmur. It was considered that he had prolapsed a mitral valve leaflet. Some months later he suffered further discomfort. His diastolic murmur increased, and it was assumed that the remaining leaflet had prolapsed. This was confirmed by echocardiography. He was subjected to open heart surgery, which I recorded on video and still retain. During the operation the papillary muscles were clearly shown to be very eroded, with the leaflets and the chordae tendineae free in the bloodstream. Another striking feature was the rotary gyration of the heart at each beat, presumably due to the reflux of blood through the incompetent mitral valve. After the new valve was inserted and the heart started beating, again the absence of gyration was apparent. He currently remains fit and well.

No. 4. M08, DOB 1962. Diagnosed 1988. This young man was first seen March 1988, when there was a mild epidemic of coxsackie B virus group 3 illness. He had a sixteenfold rise in coxsackie B virus group 3 and a positive ELISA IgM. By May he had a positive IgG together with a positive VP1 and his serological titers rose thirty-two-fold. His initial symptoms were of the usual gripping and boring pain, which he described as feeling as if someone had thrust a knife into his posterior left chest and was turning it around. He collapsed on three occasions, and his father on one occasion thought he was dead. He was referred to the hospital, but, as nothing was evident, he was referred for psychiatric advice. I have had several similar cases and believe they were due to dysrythmic attacks from the early myocarditis. As shown in this chapter, some indeed did die. This patient's ECGs became quite abnormal, with ventricular extrasystoles, and a "toxic Wenckebach" type of rhythm when the PR interval suddenly became pathologically long. He was started on IgG 750 mg by intramuscular infusion, initially once a week. After a few weeks it was given twice weekly. His ECGs normalized (see Figure 2.6a), and he became quite well. After several months of this treatment it was found that his VP1 was consistently negative, and it was decided to cease IgG therapy. Unhappily his symptoms recurred, and his ECG again showed the same features as at the commencement of the illness (Figure 2.6b). His VP1 again became positive. This was shown in a case discussed in the treatise by Rachel Jenkins and Professor Mowbray (1991). Unhappily, he did not wish to recommence IgG, and his ECG remains very abnormal with a Wenckebach phenomenon and runs of atrial tachycardia. Unfortunately, there have been runs of ventricular tachycardia also, and he has felt faint at times but has not collapsed. Nodal ablation is being considered, but at this writing I am not totally happy about it, as it would not necessarily stop the runs of ventricular tachycardia. Thus the question remains whether IgG infusions would have prevented this present recurrence.

Female Patients

No. 1. F05, DOB 1949. Diagnosed 1979. Died 1982. This patient had a typical viral illness with serial titers of coxsackie B group 4 rising to 1/512. All other titers were normal. She had positive ELISA

FIGURE 2.6a. M08, ECG L2, After IgG Treatment

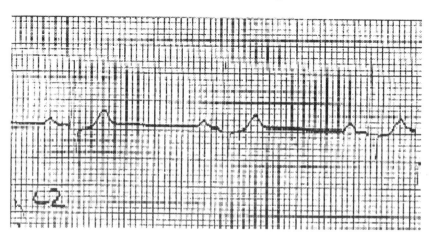

FIGURE 2.6b. M08, ECG L2, Recurring Wenckebach After Cessation of IgG Treatment

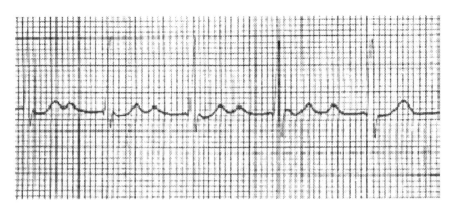

IgM and IgG, but no culture was attempted. She had symptoms of breathlessness and chest oppression, but investigation in a hospital yielded no evidence of angina. Her serial ECGs showed the changes of acute myocarditis, but she gradually remitted and was soon back to her chores. All went well for a year or so, and her ECG became normal. However, she had a minor relapse but seemed to recover until, without any warning one Saturday afternoon, outside her home she collapsed next to her car. On arrival I found that the patient had died. I had not seen her for some time and referred her for autopsy. The postmortem examination demonstrated myocarditis.

No. 2. F06, DOB 1937. Diagnosed 1974. Died 1987. This woman, whom I had known for twenty years and for whom I delivered her only child, had a marked viral illness of the Bornholm type, and at the time of the illness she had two epileptic attacks. This resolved in weeks, but afterward she developed a perimyocarditis with the usual ECG changes and a pericardial friction rub. This took about two years to resolve and the ECG to normalize, and she remained fairly well for years and was active and without pain. Her serial titers of coxsackie B group 4 at that time rose to 1/512 and also B5 to 1/64 and, more unusual, her B6 rose to 1/64. No other significant titers were found. The high titers remained for a matter of months and then fell. She also had a positive ELISA IgM and IgG and a positive culture during the initial illness. Like others, she remitted and remained well for years, but in

1986, she had another recurrence and her titers rose again to a similar height. The ECG varied from time to time but tended to show slight prolongation of the Q-T interval and marked S-T depression with varying biphasic or inverted T waves. She was referred to a hospital, where it was considered that she might have angina. Thus, she took an exercise tolerance test and her heart rate rose to a reported 179 beats per minute, but she had no pain. She told me that she had to abandon the test because of breathlessness and fatigue in her limbs. She was listed for isotope examination but had absolutely no evidence of angina, though the exercise tolerance test had left her feeling desperately exhausted for all of that and the following day. On that day I was visiting the young man in the hospital who also had a viral myocarditis and had a successful transplant. On returning, I was informed that this woman had collapsed at her tea table, and a partner had been called to the home but found she had died. On autopsy the postmortem examination revealed a cardiomyopathy.

Cardiomyopathy Group

Male Patients

No 1. M09, DOB 1920. Diagnosed 1973. Died 1974. This fifty-four-year-old man was well until he suddenly developed a cough and respiratory distress. Subsequent investigations with X rays showed a viral pneumonitis. He recovered in weeks, but his serial titers showed a rise in coxsackie B group 4 of more than 1/512, and he also had ELISA IgM and IgG and a positive stool culture. His CH50 was 48 and his C3 98. In the following months he began to be breathless, and the apical heart sounds moved to the left axillary line without any murmurs. His ECG showed a developing dialated cardiomyopathy, and he was given anticoagulants. He appeared to improve a little but remained short of breath, with poor cardiac function. He was found dead on the bathroom floor one Saturday morning. An autopsy was performed in this case and states, "the heart is enlarged and weighs 450 grams and there is localized dilatation of the ventricle posteriorly. The right ventricle appears normal. The coronary arteries showed atheromatus deposits but there was no evidence of any recent infarction." This case probably shows the results of multifactorial pathology considered earlier, as evidenced in the work of Professor Loria (1986b, 1988), in which the combination of virus and cholesterol were synergistic agents in the production of heart disease mortality.

No. 2. M10, DOB 1936. Diagnosed 1968. Died 1972. This man presented with an acute viral illness, was short of breath, and had general malaise. His serial titers of coxsackie B group 4 also rose to 1/512, and he had positive ELISA IgM and IgG tests performed, but no culture was attempted. His CH50 complement test fell to 46 and his C3 was 88. He was hospitalized under the excellent care of my colleague Dr. R. Gold. He had gross changes, apparent on serial ECGs, confirming a cardiomyopathy. Later, X rays confirmed a dilated cardiomyopathy (as shown in Figure 2.7a and Figure 2.7b). His subsequent course over a few years was rather chronic and unremitting, and he died due to congestive heart failure. No postmortem was done as the diagnosis and outcome were predictable. The question arises once again as to what would happen today in such a case. If this occurred now, would he have a heart transplant to spare his life? I re-

FIGURE 2.7a. M10's X Ray

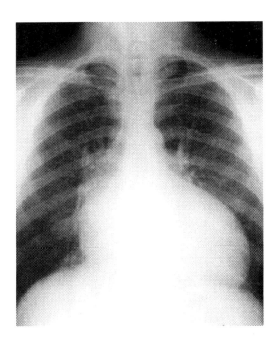

FIGURE 2.7b. M10's ECG

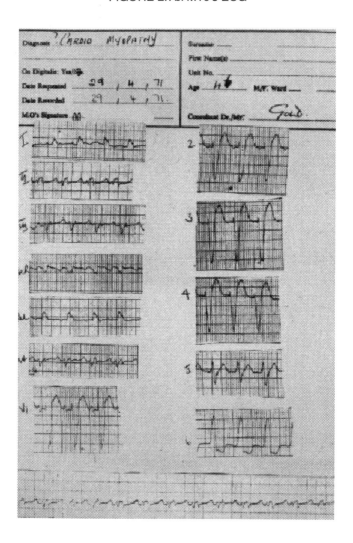

fer to two cases from more recent years in which this has been done, though one case, cited in the next section, might have been saved if the transplant had been performed earlier.

No. 3. M11, DOB 1927. Diagnosed 1973. Died 1974. This man came from abroad and was the father in Family 01 in Chapter 4, whose daughter suffered from a congenital type of amyotrophy, from which she died at the age of fifteen. Prior to visiting England, he and his wife had both had viral illnesses. At the time, he complained of chest pain and had apparently collapsed twice, possibly due to a dysrhythmia. He had been admitted to a hospital and was discharged, as it was thought that he had recovered. His medication on discharge was Lanoxin 0.125 mg and aldactone 1 daily. He was thoroughly investigated by my colleague, Dr. H. A. Dewar, and eventually discharged to my care. X rays showed him to have an enlarged heart (Figure 2.8), although he was not in failure, and his ECG was very abnormal with widely inverted T waves, frequent ventricular extrasystoles, and partial atrioventricular heart block (as shown in Figure 2.9).

His serological titers of coxsackie B virus showed a thirty-two-fold rise in group 2 and sixteenfold rise in group 4, and his wife had a similar rise in group 2. His ELISA IgM and IgG were both positive, his CH50 was 48, and his C3 was 96. As stated in the history given for his wife, they returned to their home abroad, where his baby girl was born, and subsequently he collapsed and died. Stained sections of his myocardium were sent to me and are still preserved. They show the classical changes seen in these cases of cardiomyopathy.

FIGURE 2.8. M-11's X Ray

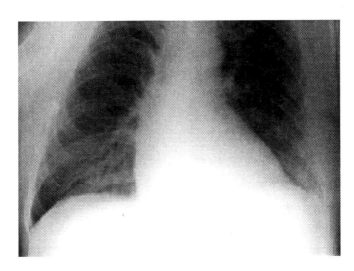

FIGURE 2.9. M11's ECG

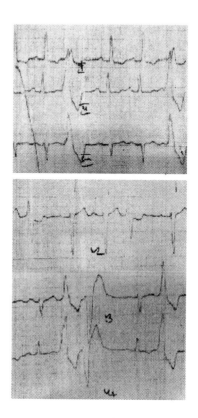

Female Patients

No. 1. F07, DOB 1928. Diagnosed 1978. Died 1981. This patient had a history similar to the others with the typical ECG changes, particularly of the T wave abnormalities mentioned earlier. Serial serological titers of coxsackie B group 4 again showed a rise to 1/512, without any other significant findings. Initially she had a positive ELISA IgM and later IgG. However, as with others, the T wave abnormalities varied from lead to lead from day to day, suggesting a changing pattern of repolarization. She gradually recovered and apparently became well, but the ECG remained abnormal and her heart showed signs of enlargement. I was particularly unhappy about these changes as she was also breathless on exertion, but without any anginal pain. The family, for her sake, moved to a smaller house but they had not been there very long before she had heart failure and died. Hospital admission and checkup had confirmed the findings, but at her age the question of transplant was never raised. The postmortem report stated:

> The heart (565 grams) showed gross left ventricular hypertrophy on external examination. The left ventricle when dissected weighed 362 grams and the right ventricle 60 grams. . . . Occasional areas of patchy interstitial fibrosis were scattered throughout the ventricles . . . and there was no evidence of recent or remote myocardial infarction. . . . Microscopic examination: Sections taken from the left ventricle showed very marked fibre hypertrophy and patchy interstitial fibrosis in the absence of inflammation or infarction. In the septum especially, there was fibre disarray with branching and the overall appearances were entirely in keeping with a diagnosis of hypertrophy obstructive cardiomyopathy. . . . The valves appeared intrinsically normal and the coronary arteries showed virtually no atheromatus disease and no evidence of thrombotic occlusion. The aorta showed minimal atheroma.

No. 2. F08, DOB 1932. Diagnosed 1964. Died 1986. This patient had a long and chronic illness, commencing with a pneumonitis and later a myocarditis and some dysrythmias. Her serial titers of coxsackie B group 4 were 1/1024 and of group 5 were 1/32. She also had positive ELISA IgM and later IgG, and her CH50 was 88 and her C3 78 in the early stages. She had an apparent remission from the acute stage but was never well and, although followed up by myself and hospital investigation, no more information was forthcoming, though there was a suggestion of endocarditis. This was never proven, but the heart size gradually but relentlessly increased to a fairly gross dilated cardiomyopathy. The apical sounds of the heart were maximum in the posterior axillary line, which was confirmed several times on X ray. Two years later, she had a stroke due to an embolus and subsequently received anticoagulants. This has been reported in other series of assumed endocarditis. However, her condition thereafter gradually deteriorated, and she died from chronic congestive heart failure.

Myocarditis with Other Syndromes

Male Patients

No 1. M12, DOB 1938. Diagnosed 1972. Died 1989. This man, whom I saw late one evening in 1972 as a private patient, gave a history suggestive of a previous viral illness. On examination it was found that he had a tachycardia with a variable pericardial friction rub and his ECGs were abnormal, in keeping with a diagnosis of myopericarditis (see Figure 2.10a). His serial coxsackie B group 4 titers rose to 1/1024

FIGURE 2.10a. M12's ECG

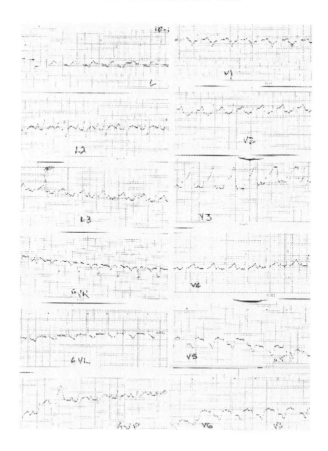

and to 1/128 for group 5. He also had a positive ELISA IgM, but again it was too late for culture. After a few appointments he ceased to visit, and it was assumed that he had returned to his native country in Africa. This apparently was not so, as he had been going to the hospital. I had no further news of him until he was brought urgently to my surgery one night in 1989. On that occasion he had gross dyspnea, a 4 cm juglar venous pressure (JVP) and, on abdominal examination, there was a large hepatomegally. His apical sounds were in the left posterior axillary line, and he had a very gross systolic and diastolic murmur, which was not obvious when auscultating the front of his chest. He was urgently referred to the hospital and admitted the following day and shortly afterward was given a cardiac transplant. The microscopy of the explanted heart showed gross changes compatible with the previous diagnosis of viral myocarditis (as shown in Figure 2.10b). Unfortunately, he did not live many months before he died, presumably due to a rejection of the transplanted heart. This case is listed because of the fact that he died not from the cardiomyopathy, but from presumed autoimmune rejection.

No. 2. M13, DOB 1947. Diagnosed 1978. Died 1986. This man had a very typical and severe attack of Bornholm disease lasting days, during which he lay on the drawing room floor curled up in front of a

FIGURE 2.10b. Microscopy of Explanted Heart—Viral Myocarditis

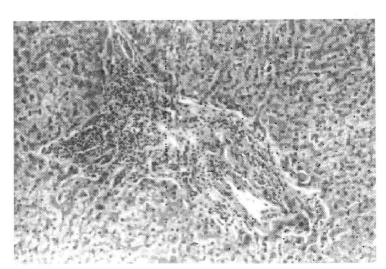

fire and, like so many others, had to have several injections of morphine daily to help him tolerate the pain. Many weeks later he became breathless and had a very typical ECG showing signs of a rather severe myocarditis but without dysrhythmia. He also showed marked signs of encephalitis, but the cardiac component appeared to be the most dramatic feature of his illness at the time. His serological titers of the coxsackie B group were as follows: group 1/64; group 2/64; group 3/128; group 4 > 1/1000; group 5/64. He had positive ELISA IgM and IgG and a positive VP1. Unfortunately, this illness lasted a long while, and he had to give up his work and sell his home as he could not afford the mortgage. After a long illness he recovered sufficiently to buy a grocery business, which his wife largely managed. During this time he had a relatively minor relapse but recovered. He later sold the business and went into the taxi trade. Quite suddenly he developed headaches and within very few months had optical congestive fundal signs suggesting raised intracranial pressure. I referred him for further neurological investigation, which confirmed the raised intracranial pressure, but sadly he died from a glioma of the brain. There have been seventeen cerebral tumors in this series, following viral encephalitis, which occurred many years after the original viral infection in which encephalitis was a result.

Female Patients

No. 1. F09, DOB 1924. Diagnosed 1980. Died 1984. This patient also commenced with viral pneumonitis and later myocarditis, without dysrhythmias but with the typical ECG changes of myocarditis. Her serial titers of coxsackie B virus, groups 3 and 5, were 1/512, with respiratory syncytial virus titers of 1/64. She also had positive ELISA IgM and IgG responses confirmed in two laboratories. She experienced unremitting decline. She developed a stenosing alveolitis after about two years, which no doubt compounded her congestive heart failure (CHF). All the treatment for CHF and steroids for her pulmonary condition only gave some symptomatic relief and, like one or two others in this series, she died due to a combination of the two syndromes. Three males likewise had identical illnesses with the same outcome.

No. 2. F10, DOB 1948. Diagnosed 1980. Died 1982. This young woman illustrates the multifarious problems that may beset patients with virus-induced illness. Initially she had cervicitis, which yielded papilloma virus and was treated. This did not cause problems. Later she had a coxsackie B group 4 infection with titers rising to 1/512 and to 1/64 in groups 2 and 3. She also had positive ELISA IgM and IgG. She initially had a Bornholm disease-type illness, and it is interesting that her mother developed an identical illness at the same time. This patient went on to develop a perimyocarditis, evidenced by a pericardial friction rub and abnormal ECGs. Later she developed a general vasculitis with an ESR of 70, and it was thought (erroneously) that she might have deep-vein thrombosis in one leg. However, I examined the venous flow in the popliteal fossa by Doppler scan and all was normal. There was a strong difference of opinion concerning this as well as the rationale for treatment. In the end, anticoagulants were given, though I was very unhappy about it as there was no sign of endocarditis or emboli. Subsequently, after a matter of a week or two, she suddenly collapsed, and while I was visiting elsewhere she was taken to a hospital and died. At autopsy the cause of death was shown to be a large brain hemorrhage. The question here is whether the hemorrhage was due to vasculitis per se, or was it compounded by the anticoagulants? Her death was never known to her mother who, as with others in this series, had developed retroperitoneal cancer, probably as a sequel to the virus-induced sick cell syndrome from previous pancreatitis. Sadly, she died only a few days after her daughter.

No. 3. F11, DOB 1951. Diagnosed 1972. Died 1989. This patient developed a febrile illness with acute chest pain, which progressed to general myositis. She was so crippled that she had to have elbow crutches. Her ECG showed the typical changes of myocarditis (see Figure 2.11). Her serological titers showed a rise to > 1/512 for coxsackie B group 4 and also a sixteenfold rise for coxsackie B group 5. Her ELISA IgM became positive as did her IgG later. Subsequently she developed pancreatitis, which resulted in diabetes mellitus. She had a young daughter who, years later, had an attack of Bornholm disease with similar high titers of the same groups of coxsackievirus. The mother was seen by general physicians, diabetes specialists, and rheumatologists and is a good example of the danger that specialists will not recognize the pleomorphic picture of multiple syndromes of com-

FIGURE 2.11. F11's ECG

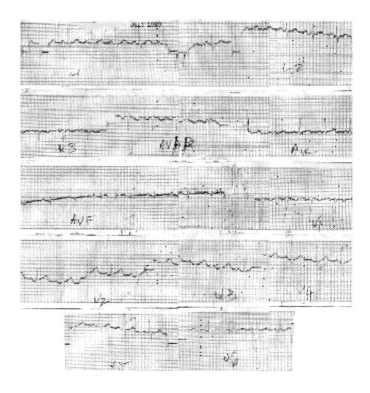

mon etiology. As in other cases, it was not possible to get colleagues really interested in the cardiology of this patient. In addition, some thought that she was making heavy weather of her muscle pain and thought that she was psychologically depressed. In July 1989, she had an exacerbation of her symptoms with the same oppressive chest pain and a marked PFR. Her ECG at that time was not alarming but showed body tremor, with the inferior leads showing a splintering effect. She battled on with her bodily symptoms and was supported by a very caring husband. On a bleak Tuesday morning in November 1989, I was called by her husband, as she felt so unwell and breathless. I found her confined to bed, dyspneic, and displaying all the symptoms of her previous cardiac illness. Fortunately I had taken my ECG recorder with me, anticipating some such event. She had not collapsed but had a

PFR, and the ECG (Figure 2.12) showed significant changes. At this point she was talking normally and apologizing for calling the doctor, to which I just had time to tell her once again that it was a privilege to attend her and try to help. She then had a sudden collapse and, as with some others, her eyes simply rolled upward and she died due to a dysrhythmic cardiac arrest. I insisted on an autopsy, which confirmed the diagnosis of cardiomyopathy.

FIGURE 2.12. F11's Second ECG

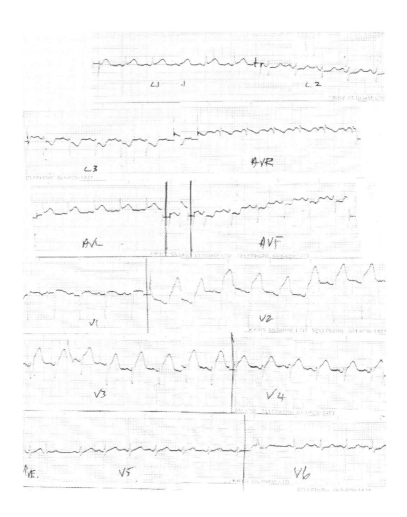

No. 4. F12, DOB 1937. Diagnosed 1974. This woman was a nurse in a local hospital and, during 1974, there was a local outbreak of coxsackie-mediated illnesses. She presented with acute myocarditis with malaise, chest oppression, and breathlessness. Her titers of coxsackie B were as follows: group 1 = 1/8; group 2 = 1/256; group 3 = 1/32; group 4 = 1/128; group 5 = 1/8; group 6 = 1/8; and also a positive ELISA IgM, IgG, and IgA response. Her complement CH50 fell to 36 percent, the C3 was 93, and the virus was isolated in her case. ECG examinations were performed on many subsequent occasions and show the changing patterns described in others with frequent ventricular ectopic beats (Figure 2.13). She made a slow recovery but developed antithyroid antibodies, though she never became myxedematous. This has oc-

FIGURE 2.13. F12's ECG

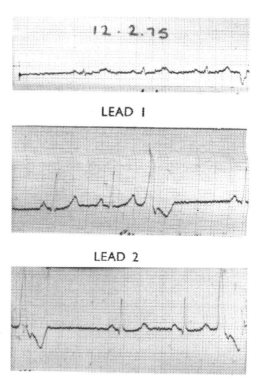

LEAD 1

LEAD 2

LEAD 3

curred in 20 percent in this series of virus-mediated illness and also in Dr. Irving Spurr's cases more recently (personal communication). She then developed a marked scapular muscle dystrophy, as others have done. It was not due to disuse atrophy and gradually remitted. She also had mildly prominent eyes but was not thyrotoxic. She was referred to the hospital for a muscle biopsy that I had arranged and intended to send to Dr. Archard at Charing Cross for polymerase chain reaction (PCR) examination for possible viral sequences. However, a young doctor who saw her was obviously bemused by the apparent exophthalmos and prescribed carbimazole. I was not informed about this at the time, but within two weeks I was called to her home to find her bordering on myxedematous coma. This remitted as soon as the drug was withdrawn. Unhappily, the muscle biopsy was never performed due to the ensuing illness and the mismanagement at the time of admission. The acute episode settled after many months and the myopathy remitted after a year or two. She then went on to develop a typical rheumatoid illness that caused severe deformities and has required multiple joint prostheses. This case illustrates the autoimmune sequences that can develop after an enteroviral infection.

Perimyocarditis

Female Patients

No. 1. F13, DOB 1927. Diagnosed 1985. This woman had typical perimyocarditis with chest pain in the lower sternal area and pain in the outer border of the left arm. Her coxsackie B titers were more than 1/512 for group 4, with positive ELISA IgG and IgG. Her ECG showed all the typical changes, and she had the usual marked pericardial friction rub. This took several months to abate before she returned to normal health, although she had T wave inversion in limb leads and lateral chest leads. She had a further exacerbation in 1985, which remitted. Following a flu vaccination in 1994, she had a more severe exacerbation with the same symptoms. Her ECG (Figures 2.14 and 2.15) demonstrates the changes that occurred, and echocardiography confirmed the pericardial effusion. This episode took about three months to pass, and the remarkable outcome has been the restoration of upright T waves for the first time in ten years. The reason for this change is currently being discussed and is still sub judice.

FIGURE 2.14. F13's ECG, 1985

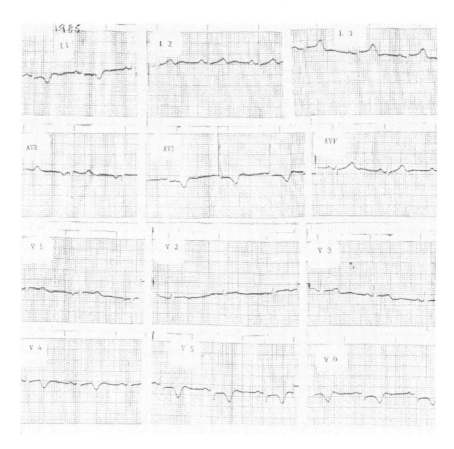

SUMMARY

The case reports make no reference to early treatment. This raises questions as well as observations. Perhaps the use of IgG in myocarditis is a serious consideration. For varying reasons, this was not used in any of the cases mentioned in Group 5 earlier. The question, therefore, would be whether a fatal outcome could have been averted if IgG had been given. Case M07 does demonstrate the results of this therapy and also the unhappy results of too-early withdrawal. My colleague, Dr. R. Gold, has also used IgG with success and has shown that in case of relapse it can be effective. The raison d'être will be discussed in Chapter 9.

FIGURE 2.15. F13's ECG, 1995

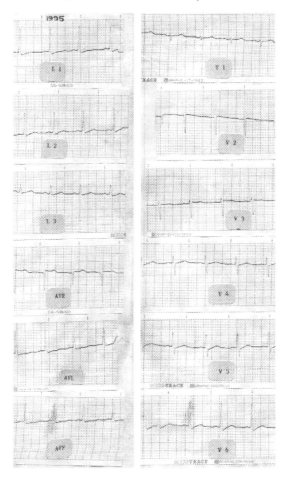

Out of the 1,780 cases of virus-mediated illness stored on a computer, these are but a few of those who presented initially with a cardiac syndrome. They are not particularly selected as the "worst cases," although many come from Group 5 (i.e., those who died), and thus the autopsy results were available. As shown, this did not exclude other organic illness of similar etiology.

The IgG and IgM tests were all by the ELISA method and confirmed in two laboratories independently.

The histories have been condensed to mere factual evidence of virus-mediated sequential illness. Once again I would remark that these are not just "cases" but are human beings in a family setting, well known, cared for, and followed up over four decades. In some of the families, other members had an illness due to the same strain of virus but without a cardiac consequential illness. The case histories are extremely concise, but hundreds of ECGs and serial virological titers were performed over the years. Many are still available, though it would be repetitive and wearisome to try to publish them.

Chapter 3
Central Nervous System Effects
of Viral Origin

INTRODUCTION

As will be shown, CNS effects range from congenitally acquired syndromes to those that occur later in life. The various symptoms are related to the function of the area affected, in these cases after an initial or ongoing viral infection. Generally the listed cases have been divided up into groups, showing the resulting effects on the higher centers and also the spinal cord. The total number of cases is 678, of which 221 are male and 457 are female. This shows the greater proportion of females in all cases where central nervous system effects occurred.

Since the lower parts of the brain are affected in many cases in this series, it may be wise to briefly review the functions of these parts. The hypothalamus itself is the chief caretaker of the basic biological needs of the body, including growth, metabolic rate, blood pressure, heart and respiration rate, gut activity including appetite, varying gland secretions, and control of the RBC circulating population and blood sugar, as well as sleep and emotional reactions. The posterior area by and large controls sympathetic activity, while the anterior portion controls parasympathetic activity. This control affects the entire organic system, and thus some effects that may appear remote may have their origin in alterations in hypothalamic function.

Irritable bowel syndrome (IBS), which occurred in certain cases, is a good example and is probably multifactorial. It is controlled by both neuronal and endocrine factors. The neuronal factors operate through pathways involving the cortex, hypothalamus, and brain stem as well as intrinsic and extrinsic pathways in the gut itself. This activity is a good example of what can occur in muscle, for gut muscle has two rhythms, one at 3 cycles per minute (c/m) and the other at about 8 c/m. The bowel is controlled mainly by the dominant rhythm. If the 3 c/m rhythm is dominant then IBS results. The rhythm can be heard with the stethoscope or measured by ultrasound and is what I call "boiling bowel syndrome." In the hypothalamus, stimulation of the posterior area results in a rise in adrenalin, blood pressure and respiratory rate as well as a concomitant inhibition of gut activity, appetite (causing anorexia), and bladder function. Moreover, in both experimental animals and humans "rage syndrome" can be generated as well as spontaneous pain. Stimulation of the anterior area, on the other hand, causes increase in appetite, and increased gut and bladder activity, as well as proctalgia, vaginismus, diminished blood pressure and heart rate, and somnolence. In an enraged bull, an electrode implanted in this area, when activated by remote control, will cause the animal to be quite placid. The author has shown that the effects of monoamine oxidase inhibitors, if enhanced by eating cheese, exert their toxic effects by posterior hypothalamic stimulation, which may result in hypertensive encephalopathy, as seen in a case that was published years ago in the *Newcastle Medical Journal.*

The hypothalamus can also be affected by certain heavy metals and virus infections, and the effects may persist long after the initiating factor has been withdrawn. Thus an imbalance of hypothalamic function, by stimulation or inhibition of either the anterior or posterior area, can result in a wide range of symptoms that may be assumed to be psychological in origin. Also, depending on the area affected, a variety of symptoms may be seen in any single patient. The hypothalamic effects may also be mediated by neurohormonal pathways via other glands, that is the pituitary and pineal.

The functions of the limbic system may be briefly summarized as follows:

1. *Thalamus.* The communication link between the body's afferent reflexes and the cortex.
2. *Hypothalamus.* Generally regulates autonomic processes and analyzes both afferent and efferent impulses. As a result, endorphins are secreted here.
3. *Amygdala.* The name refers to its almond shape. It is generally referred to as the aggression center and initiates sudden behavioral responses.

4. *Hippocampus*. The name refers to its seahorse shape. It is considered to deal with olfactory and visceral sense, e.g., taste. It also harbors immediate and short-term memory sensations.
5. *Cerebellum*. This well-known section is linked to higher cortical mechanisms via the limbic system and thus correlates autonomic functions, e.g., balance, with higher conscious functions.

The pituitary is connected by the neurohypophysial stalk to the pars posterior commissurae anterioris and by a portal circulation to the anterior lobe. The secreted neuroactive substances are profuse—nearly forty of which are known already. They range from the angiotensins through oxytocins, vasopressins, corticotropin releasing hormone (CRH), glucagon, dopamine, etc., to growth hormone-releasing factor (GHRF), acetylcholine and prolactin. Prolactin is known to reflect the 5-hydroxytryptamine (5-HT) mechanism, and in myalgic encephalomyelitis there is an up-regulation of the 5-HT system. This can be measured simply by taking an early morning blood sample to measure prolactin, giving 60 mg buspirone, and measuring the serum levels one hour later, when there will be as much as a 400 percent rise in some patients compared to levels found in normal or endogenously depressed patients, in whom the rise is less than 200 percent.

The pineal gland is likewise involved in the neurohormnal process. It is innervated by a postganglionic supply from the superior cervical ganglia. This chain is regulated by impulses from the suprachiasmatic nucleus (SCN) of the hypothalamus. This nucleus receives impulses from the retina and the retinohypothalamic tract. This nerve supply to the pineal gland from the postganglionic sympathetic supply travels via noradrenergic fibers, and all functions are mediated by beta-adrenergic receptors. It does not share the blood-brain barrier of the rest of the higher cortical system. Exposure to bright light at certain times can suppress melatonin secretion and arrest the circadian rhythms.

The hormones involved in the neurohormonal process include the amines, such as noradrenaline, serotonin, histamine, melatonin, dopamine, luteinizing hormone-releasing hormone (LH-RH), thyrotropin-releasing hormone (TRH), somatostatin, and the inhibitory neurotransmitter gamma-aminobutyric acid (GABA). During darkness, melatonin secretion is highest and serotonin low. Sympathetic or hypoglycemic stress can increase melatonin activity, and an increase of melatonin will induce a lowering of plasma luteinizing hormone (LH) and growth hormone (GH) levels. It also causes sleepiness and increase in REM (rapid eye movement) sleep as seen on the EEG.

This may have a bearing on the fact that some ME cases, as well as one case that was studied in a congenitally brain-damaged man, find bright light uncomfortable and darkness more tolerable, and yet do not sleep at night but develop the owl syndrome. The mechanism is not totally clear, but probably the desire for darkness is more a symptom of the underlying abnormality than a cause of it. In some cases a change in urine specific gravity (SG) and the volume of urine excreted has also been noticed, and a simple water dilution test was found helpful in defining it. This test is simple and consists of measuring the SG of the first morning sample at, say, 9 a.m. Two liters of water are then taken within half an hour, and the urine passed during the next three hours is collected. The normal person will pass 80 percent of that imbibed and the affected patient will pass only 40 percent to 60 percent, but the SG is often low. This presumably reflects the variation of nocturnal secretion of antidiuretic hormone.

PAIN

Pain is a subjective phenomenon, perceived by the higher brain centers. It may be a specific sensation coming from pain receptors, or from end organs that have free nerve endings of naked axis cylinders, forming a terminal arborization of uninsulated fibrils among the other cells, as for instance in the cornea or tympanic membrane. In these specialized end organs, apart from their normal function of either seeing or hearing, the only other form of sensibility is for pain. They are unlike the ordinary receptor end organs for temperature, touch, etc., which have well-developed laminated capsules that insulate the nerve fibers from other tissues. The centers for unlocalized feeling are not in the cortex but in the thalamus. Thus, central pain, which is separate from peripheral pain, be it due to specific nerve end organ stimulation or to naked axial insult, has its origin, as stated, in the thalamus.

A vascular lesion in the thalamus can cause so-called hemiplegia dolorosa which can be exacerbated by sudden bright light, noise, or intense odors. In addition, normal feeling is affected and may account for the severe sensitivity in some cases, where touching or stroking a limb or the skin evokes a painful response. Some patients with ME describe feelings of "pins and needles," itching, flushing, and "electric feelings" similar to faradic stimulation. These feelings are most likely of thalamic origin. One seventeen-year-old patient described this as "trillions of little pains." She also had episodes of involuntary and precipitate micturition, which are known to occur in some thalamic disorders.

OPTIC SIGNS

Some patients with ME also complain of focusing difficulties. The optic tract runs backward to the primary optic center in the pulvinar portion of the optic thalamus and thence to the calcarine area of the cortex via the retrobulbar tract. The reflex centers that control pupillary contraction for accommodation are sometimes affected in this condition. The nucleus of the third or occulomotor nerve lies in the gray matter of the floor of the aqueduct of the midbrain. It is composed of small nuclei as follows:

1. The dorsilateral nucleus (concerned with upward movements)
2. The ventromedial nucleus (concerned with downward movements)
3. The central nucleus (concerned with convergence)
4. The Edinger-Westphal nucleus (situated more dorsally in the gray matter of the midbrain and concerned with the sphincter pupillae and ciliary muscles)
5. The caudate central nucleus (this probably functions with the Edinger-Westphal nucleus)

The ciliary ganglion is the size of a pinhead and is situated in fat between the eye and the lateral rectus muscle. Its preganglionic fibers are derived from the Edinger-Westphal nucleus and travel to the ganglion; they are parasympathetic motor fibers. The sympathetic root comes from the superior cervical ganglion and traverses the ciliary ganglion. Its action is to cause miosis of the pupil, while the fibers from the third nerve cause mydriasis. If carefully examined, some cases of ME will be found to have a lack of pupillary contraction to accommodation with preservation of the light reflex, a condition the reverse of the Argyll Robertson pupil (Purves-Stewart).

Abnormalities are recorded as occurring in cases of chronic encephalitis and also in postdiphtheritic toxic neuritis. Most recently, in 1992, they were confirmed as occurring in ME by Sadun (1991). In the series here described they occurred in about 2 percent of cases, and it was more often the younger group who complained of this focusing difficulty. Examination of the eyes usually showed a rather dilated pupil, which contracted poorly to light and scarcely at all to accommodation. They can easily be recorded on videotape, which has been done in this series. Vertical movements of the eyeballs known as curtseying but not hippus occurs in some cases also. The pupil, after contracting for accommodation, fails to maintain it and begins to dilate. These physiological abnormalities could well account for some symptoms experienced by patients who suffer from ME. In some cases, if examined carefully, the central retinal veins will be found to have a "cuffing," which is probably due to cerebrospinal fluid (CSF) infiltration between the vein and the meningeal reflections onto the vessel. Similar infiltration of Virchow-Robin spaces in the brain is considered by Mena and colleagues (p. 432) to be the reason for the so-called unidentified bright objects (UBOs) seen on MRI scans in patients with ME.

HISTORY

The CNS syndromes in this series followed an onset that was merely a flulike type of illness, involving either the respiratory or gastrointestinal tracts with or without pain, vomiting, or diarrhea. In some, glandular involvement was found. The initial illness could vary from mild to severe and when examined, in many cases, petechiae were seen on the posterior pharyngeal wall, which extended down to the respiratory or gastric mucosa. The gastrointestinal pathology caused effects similar to the so-called phlegmonous gastritis described in Chapter 5. The vomit often looked "gravylike" and in the case of an eleven-year-old boy resulted in a continuing hematemesis, and he had to be transfused.

Again, a pneumonic syndrome is prodromal in some; this is a "pneumonitis" that is demonstrated on X ray and may mimic miliary

TB. However, on other occasions an acute illness manifests itself by severe pleurodynia, anginoid or abdominal pain, and sometimes syncope. These symptoms may remit and return in three or four days in about 60 percent of cases, and in another 20 percent a third attack even worse than the first may occur. However, if recovery is full and complete within three to six months, patients are listed in Group 1 and the cases are kept on file. It is noteworthy that 20 percent of Group 1 have a second occurrence, perhaps years later. In these cases also the symptoms may remit entirely or go on to systemic organ disturbance, as outlined in other chapters.

Disturbance is often gradual, the patient not feeling fully recovered. The symptoms may be cardiac, renal, pancreatic, or, as in this chapter, occur in the central nervous system. As an example, one case involved a young women in whom adrenal changes took place, which was thought to be a type of Addison's disease. This subsequently proved to be incorrect, for steroids were of no help. She was subsequently mainly confined to her room and had muscle softening and wasting, with severe leg jitter, anomia, and all the other signs of ME.

However, the illness may affect the neurovegative function, as outlined previously, or the lower motor neurons. The thermoregulatory mechanism is recognized by the patient having episodes of hot and cold feelings, and relatives often notice the color changes in the face. Sweating, cramps, painful muscle groups, and sometimes wasting may occur. Two cases, a man and a woman, suffered gross humeroscapular wasting that later remitted.

Palpitations with labile blood pressure and faint feelings are not uncommon, as is the feeling of "inward trembling" and, in a few, labile personality changes. In the era around 1950 to 1960, we had some cases of acute schizophrenia following a viral illness that necessitated hospitalization, but most of these recovered without relapse.

Focusing difficulties and intolerance of noise are fairly frequent. In a small number, epileptic fits may occur in the acute stage and may recur later; on the other hand, a syndrome similar to narcolepsy has been observed in the author's series. These patients, however, do not lose consciousness but have akinetic lapses in which, though aware of their surroundings, they are unable to move or communicate. These attacks usually last only minutes.

A reversal of sleep pattern occurs in some. These patients will not sleep at night but feel tired during the day and, like the owl and other nocturnal animals, are awake during the hours of darkness. This phenomenon has been graded depending on the time sleep usually occurs.

Following the acute or relapsing illness, pleomorphic symptoms may emerge that baffle the patient and the physician alike. They may be a part of the hypothalamic syndrome or in some cases be due to concomitant infection of another organ. One does not exclude the other and, as shown elsewhere in this series, 30 percent of the CNS cases had some other organ pathology due to a common etiology.

In the CNS cases, the acute case can be defined as embolic, hemorrhagic, or infective—by either bacterial or viral infection. In this series the focus is on virus-mediated syndromes. In many, however, it is often difficult to define a precise time of origin, and indeed the CNS series show the difference between insidious and chronic disease syndromes. This is reflected in the difficulty in interpreting laboratory results.

The author has shown over many years that although serological titers may be high and act as a guide to the virus as the etiological agent in the severe acute illness, they may be only moderately raised later in the chronic phase and therefore are of little help. Here the VP1 has proved consistently helpful. It should be noted that only the highest titers attained are reported in all Chapters. In all cases serial titers were done over months and sometimes years and, as noted elsewhere, the first titer may not be the highest, had titers been done earlier.

Much more sinister is the fact that in the insidious case, in which virus is harbored but is not being replicated, and when symptoms occur maybe years after the initial infection, it may be impossible to define it by ordinary serological tests. It is apparent that a number of syndromes involve a nondestructive lesion that exerts its effect, not by cell lysis, but by interfering with the physiological functions of the cell, by inhibiting membrane function, or intracellular activity by mitochondrial trauma. In these cases it may be the brain cells, the white matter, or the emerging neuronal tracts that are affected. This has been shown by several researchers and was the topic of a personal communication recently with J. K. Fazakerley, who is studying the effects of persistent viral infection on normal cell function. The late effects of virus can produce the sick cell syndrome (SCS) and cause the cell to resume an undifferentiated form. This in turn may predispose to cancer, and this could be the reason for the noted high rate of gliomas, etc., that occurred years after the initial illness in this series.

The laboratory efforts to study the effects of virus-induced disease suffer from several serious limitations. As will be discussed elsewhere, it is difficult to believe a virus has its own ability to reproduce or to mutate. This again reflects the difficulties in interpreting laboratory results.

Studying the growth of virus in cell lines in a culture medium has many drawbacks. First, the virus is confined to a particular cell line, whereas in the host there are multitudes of differing cell lines. Second, some of these cell lines are constantly changing, whereas in a culture medium this is not so. In the central nervous system, the cell lines may not change during a lifetime, whereas the cells of the circulatory system obviously are in a state of constant development and change. It can also be shown that the stage of cell development determines the pathogenicity of viral infection. Contrary to in vitro studies, in the intact host virus may be shed and can then "infect" a different cell line. This process is probably needed for the host mutation of virus. Viral studies performed in other species are a great help in defining the results of infection, but they do not completely answer the question of mutation within human families. This can result in subsequent infection and ensuing illness in another family member maybe years later, as is shown to occur in this series.

In the presumed insidious cases many questions can be posed:

1. What inhibits or initiates viral replication?
2. What determines the degree of pathogenicity? This may be linked to the previous question, and is related to viral virulence and host susceptibility or resistance.
3. What determines the recrudescence of an illness? Is it another virus, where genomic drift may occur and stimulate a latent virus, or is it a toxin, or perhaps autoimmune "failure"?

4. What determines the areas and limits of pathology, e.g., in MS where many discrete areas are apparently affected, while identical tissue in other areas or organs is apparently not affected?

SYMPTOM MIMICRY

Symptom mimicry may occur where symptoms suggest a primary organic syndrome. This is a serious hindrance to diagnosis, and only a few conditions can be mentioned here.

1. Some cases of radiculitis occurred in which a prolapsed intervertebral disc was suspected. In one case, a laminectomy was performed, which revealed a normal disc and a large inflamed posterior nerve root ganglion. See case report F19 in this chapter.
2. In the more acute stage the palpitations, respiratory distress, food aversion, and mood swings can easily be put down to a purely psychiatric disorder involving the higher cortical centers, even though the patients themselves know and state that they are not "depressed."
3. Chest pain and diaphragmatic pain, as in Bornholm disease, can, obviously, seriously mimic myocardial infarction and/or gallstone colic.
4. Eye signs occur that may include varying isolated palsies, e.g., lateral rectus palsy of one or both eyes, focusing difficulty as previously discussed, or sometimes "staring eyes" with a suggestion of exopthalmus, which may give an impression of hyperthyroidism. One patient to whom carbimazole was given on the assumption that she had hyperthyroidism was discussed previously. She became ill and was bordering on a hypothyroid coma when seen at home later. She recovered when the carbimazole was stopped, and her thyroid function tests were shown to be normal, though she had developed antithyroid antibodies, as about 20 percent of other cases do. Thyroid hormone estimation may be misleading in a very small number, as in one case of a sixty-five-year-old woman whose thyroid-stimulating hormone (TSH) suggested she had a hyperactive thyroid when, in fact, clinically she was normal and her pulse only 70 to 80 beats per minute while she was taking

thyroxine 0.1 mg three times daily. In this case there was clinical evidence of end organ receptor block to T_4, similar to the end organ block that can occur in some cases of insulin resistance.

5. The varying muscle pains, softened areas, and wasting can mimic rheumatoid arthritis or varying scapular-humeral dystrophies, etc. This can be deceptive, especially if, as in a few cases, there is a type of "liver palm" (red palms) with burning feelings, etc. These have all been reported, but when and if the illness remits, the signs cease.

These are only a few of the signs that may be misconstrued as pointing to a primary single organ dysfunction as the cause of the illness, rather than a hypothalamic regulatory dysfunction. The difficulty arises when that particular, assumed organ dysfunction is addressed, but the patient is not restored to normal health because of the persistence of the more central regulatory dysfunction. This is only a very brief summary of the difficulties that can and do arise.

Table 3.1 is a summary of the CNS syndromes noted in this series.

TABLE 3.1. CNS Syndromes Noted

Males	Cases
Total number over 4 decades	222
Encephalitis, acute	10
Encephalopathy	1
Facial palsies, etc.	5
Viral meningitis, acute	3
Midbrain syndrome, acute	11
Radiculitis	11
Labyrinthinitis	9
Myalgic encephalomyelitis	93
ME with other syndrome	57
Midbrain syndrome	11
Progressive muscle atrophy	1
Transverse myelitis syndrome	2
Parkinson syndrome	1
Guillain-Barré syndrome	1

TABLE 3.1 *(continued)*

Pseudo or possible MS	3
CNS congenital deformities	3
Females	
Total number over 4 decades	457
Encephalitis, acute	22
Encephalopathy	2
Cerebellar acute infection	2
Facial palsies, etc.	6
Viral meningitis, acute	10
Midbrain syndrome, acute	24
Radiculitis	12
Labyrinthinitis	13
Myalgic encephalomyelitis	208
ME with other syndrome	112
Midbrain syndrome	23
Transverse myelitis	3
Spasmodic retrocollis	1
Guillain-Barré syndrome	2
Pseudo or possible MS	16
Progressive muscle atrophy	1
Subacute sclerosing panencephalitis (SSPE)	3
Congenital CNS deformity	6
Spinal cord tumors	2
Brain hemorrhage	1
Epilepsy	3

The CNS congenital deformities are shown elsewhere and include early trimester agenesis of corpus callosum, septum lucidum with blindness, cavum septum pellucidum, amyelination of cortical white matter, and late-trimester brain damage.

From these tables it can be shown that, though there is an overall preponderance of females, the relative syndromes are similar in proportion. The viral etiology might be doubted by some, but if one remembers that the CNS illness was accompanied in approximately 50 percent of both male and female patients by some other syndrome ranging from cardiac, renal, or pancreatic with diabetes ensuing, to thyroid and other syndromes, then the possibility of a common etiological factor could not be ignored. Moreover, the serological tests confirmed this relationship.

ANECDOTAL CASE REPORTS

In relating these cases, it should be borne in mind that they are not presented as they would be in a hospital setting. The patients are members of families, many of whom were cared for over four decades. Hence, later illness can be related to earlier illness, not just by "taking the history" but by personal, ongoing experience. The presentations are necessarily concise, but the background experience should be kept in mind by the reader and is available, as it has all been recorded. As noted previously, the serological titers all point to a viral etiology in this group, and serial titers as well as cultures, VP1 antigen tests, etc. were all performed.

Encephalitis

F14

This woman in her fifties became acutely ill one Sunday morning. When I arrived at her home she lay on the floor in a coma, in decerebrate rigidity, and with upward deviation of the eyes to the right. Her husband had already called an ambulance, and I followed it to the hospital where she was admitted. At first it was thought that she had suffered a massive cerebral hemorrhage and no more could be done. However, the house officer accepted the clinical evidence that she had encephalitis due to a viral illness, with a probable acute vasculitic reaction. Two hundred mg of intravenous dexamethazone were prescribed and given immediately. The result was happy, for the following morning she sat up and had breakfast. Her recovery was complete.

Her serological titers that were done at the time showed a rise in coxsackie B neutralizing titers as follows: B1, 1/64; B2, 1/64; B3, 1/256; B4, 1/64; B5, 1/32; B6, 1/8. She had also a positive ELISA IgM test. She developed a myopericarditis that later remitted entirely, and later still, as with many others, she developed antithyroid antibodies. There was no change in thyroid function, however, and she remains well. Her daughter later had a baby, and a week after the initial dose of oral polio vaccine was given to the baby, the baby's mother developed a severe, acute facial palsy (polio of the face?). Her serological titers for polio group 1 rose to 1/128000, group 2 to 1/32000, and group 3 to 1/32. This case, which occurred in 1989, was reviewed in 1994, and serum samples were sent to my colleague, Professor James Mowbray, from the buffy coat of which, by PCR, he isolated poliovirus. It is of considerable interest that a clergyman who baptized a baby in the same week also developed a similar severe left-sided facial palsy, and he had a similar rise in polio titers. Neither of these cases have had any further sequelae.

Encephalopathy

F15

F15 was a young woman who was twenty weeks pregnant with a third pregnancy by the same husband. She presented at the surgery not feeling well. The fetal heartbeat was good, and her temperature and blood pressure were normal. Her urine contained a faint trace of urobilinogen. Chest and cardiovascular system (CVS) examination were normal. It was decided to reexamine her the following morning, and identical findings were elicited. Blood was taken for viral studies, which subsequently showed the following titers of coxsackie B virus: B1, 1/8; B2, 1/512; B3, 1/32; B4, 1/512; B5, 1/8; B6, 1/8. She had a positive ELISA IgM and a positive fecal culture also. She was hospitalized and observed, but the fetal heart arrested and the fetus was aborted. Sadly, she developed myocarditis and a severe headache due to encephalitis. The evidence suggested that she had a reactive generalized vasculitis. She was transferred to the intensive care unit, having also developed hepatorenal failure, and was sustained for some days, but died.

M13

This man's illness commenced with severe Bornholm disease and later a blinding headache and severe myocarditis. His titers of coxsackie B virus rose as follows: B1, 1/64; B2, 1/64; B3, 1/128; B4, 1/1024;

B5, 1/64; B6, 1/8. He had positive ELISA IgM and later IgG responses. He never lost consciousness but had signs of encephalopathy with some papilloedema, which remitted. His history is included in Chapter 2. After a stormy convalescence he recovered. The sinister sequel occurred a number of years later with the development of a glioma of the brain, which progressed rapidly, and he died.

Cerebellar Acute Ataxia

F16

In 1979 this woman, who was a nurse, had a headache and later a gross disequilibrium of a typical cerebellar pattern with the classical ataxia, but not vertigo. She was investigated in the hospital and the diagnosis confirmed. Viral titers of coxsackie B rose as follows: B1, 1/8; B2, 1/32; B3, 1/8; B4, 1/8; B5, 1/128; B6, 1/8, and she had also a positive ELISA IgM. Viral cultures from the stools were positive. She was treated with high doses of choline-dihydrogen-citrate mixture and after some months made a complete recovery.

Facial Palsies

Facial palsies have been captured on videotape and one has been alluded to earlier as case F14. Others have occurred and in several cases have reoccurred. They will be referred to in Chapter 4. It is suggested that this is an area worthy of note and that the term Bell's palsy is not adequate as it does not specify etiology. Some examples are given here.

F17

In 1979, a thirty-four-year-old female presented with a febrile viral illness, and a day or two later developed a left-sided facial palsy. Her serological titers to coxsackie B virus rose thus: B1, 1/8; B2, 1/512; B3, 1/32; B4, 1/8; and B5, 1/128. She had a positive ELISA IgM and later IgG, and also a stool culture was positive. Ten years later she had a right-sided facial palsy, and the coxsackie B virus group 2, which had fallen to normal, rose again to 1/128, and this time she also had a positive VP1 test. This was not available in 1979. It is worthy of consideration that during the first period she had two stillbirths of abnormal babies. These are reported in the section of Chapter 7 on the outcome of pregnancy in cases with coxsackie viral infection.

F18

In 1973, this thirty-year-old female, who was pregnant, presented with a febrile illness. This was a typical Bornholm disease. Her serological titers of coxsackie B rose to 1/512 for group 4, the other groups remaining normal, but her fecal culture was positive. This case is also reported in Chapter 7. The baby was born, but quickly showed signs of cardiac abnormality and died some months later from endocardial fibroelastosis. The patient's titers fell gradually to 1/32, but in 1986 she was ill and had a severe facial palsy, and there was again a rise of coxsackie B group 4 to 1/128 with a positive ELISA IgM and IgG response. This remitted and her titers fell again to 1/32, but she had a similar illness with a second facial palsy in 1988, when the same titers rose again fourfold to 1/128. This time the VP1 test was available and was strongly positive. Once again her symptoms remitted, albeit with some signs of facial muscle atrophy, but her titers again fell to 1/32. In 1989 she had a third identical recurrence; this time, titers of coxsackie B groups 2 and 4 rose to 1/128, and again her VP1 became strongly positive. Like all the others, a full viral screen did not reveal a significant rise in any other strain, including poliovirus. It may be of interest that in these years she had recurring cysts in her breasts which I aspirated, obtaining up to 100 cc of clear straw-colored fluid each time. These aspirates never showed any signs of cells or malignancy. She also had a recurring perimyocarditis and, sadly, early in 1998 collapsed and died in middle age. Postmortem demonstrated signs of a recurrent, patchy myocarditis.

M14

In 1978, this thirty-eight-year-old man presented with a febrile illness and chest pain with a pericardial friction rub. He had a fourfold rise of titer of coxsackie B virus group 4 and a positive culture. This fell over the subsequent months, and he was well until 1989, when he had a recurrent viral illness with signs of a midbrain lesion, in that he had bilateral rectus palsies, and he also developed a facial palsy. He had a fourfold rise this time in coxsackie B groups 2 and 4 and also a fourfold rise in measles virus, but he did not have any rash. His pericarditis, however, did not return. This bilateral rectus palsy is recorded on videotape. It took months for symptoms to remit, but eventually he fully recovered.

Radiculopathies

F19

This forty-year-old nurse presented in 1959 with intense burning pain in the left sciatic radiation. There was no further pain on straight leg raising, and no sensory or motor changes were found. She had had a mild febrile flulike illness. A number of investigations were performed, and she was seen by myself and an eminent neurologist who agreed that the illness was viral. Her titers of coxsackie B group 4 were raised as they were in the other cases. She refused our diagnosis and felt "something must be done," and persuaded a neurosurgeon to operate. During the operation the discs were found to be preserved, but a swollen and inflamed posterior nerve root ganglion was discovered. Afterward, the pain remained, and she insisted that something more must be done. To try to help her, the neurosurgeon offered to do a cordotomy to sever the pain tract. She accepted this, and it was duly performed. Unfortunately, this was followed by an anterior spinal artery thrombosis with resultant paresis of the lower limbs and no further amelioration of the pain. She later was transferred to another spinal unit and given an alcohol block, which resulted only in higher paresis, affecting her bladder and bowel function, but again with no lessening of the pain. Eventually, another neurosurgeon performed a leukotomy, following which she said she "still had the pain but it did not bother her so much." After several years in bed she developed bilateral, staghorn renal calculi, went into renal failure, and died. The question at the time related to the posterior nerve root ganglion and the failure of such radical operations on the spinal cord to relieve the pain. How much was this due to the local posterior nerve root ganglion inflammation, or could there have been a hypothalamic component overreacting to the pain? No clear answers were possible, but the outcome was tragic.

M15

M15 was a twenty-one-year-old male who presented initially in 1987 with Bornholm disease, and whose coxsackie B titers were as follows: B1, 1/32; B2, 1/32; B3, 1/512; B4, 1/32; B6,1/32. He had a positive ELISA IgM. This seemed to resolve, but he was ill again in 1988, and his titers of both B3 and B5 rose to 1/128, and he had again a positive ELISA IgM and IgG. This time the VP1 was done and was markedly positive. However, he developed a gross type of atrophy of the right shoulder girdle, similar to Erb atrophy (as shown in Figure 3.1). He was unlike the previous case in that he had an anterior horn type of radiculitis which mimicked that seen in poliomyelitis. This patient is also recorded on videotape, and the gross wasting is very

FIGURE 3.1. M15's Atrophy of Right Shoulder Girdle

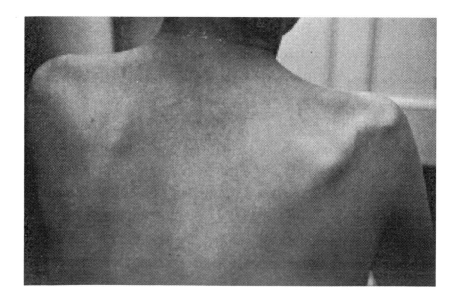

apparent. He has recovered now and is able to work. Other relations are also included in Chapter 7 as cases F36 and F37.

Labyrinthitis

F20

A nineteen-year-old girl was confined to bed after an acute minor flulike illness in 1954. She was visited and was very afraid to move, as lifting her head made her feel as if she was "shooting through the ceiling," and on lowering her head she felt as if she was "going through the floor." No nystagmus was elicited during the following days, nor did she have any vomiting. The episode lasted about a week. This was the only case I have had affecting purely the otolithic vestibular apparatus. Her coxsackie culture from a fecal specimen was positive. She made a good recovery and has never had a recurrence.

M16

M16 is a twenty-six-year-old manual worker who became ill at work in 1954. He was so unbalanced on the bus journey home that the crew thought that he was drunk. He was seen at home by myself and one of my late colleagues, who was a professor of medicine at the time. He was very interested in the syndrome. The patient had all the classic signs of labyrinthine disturbance, with violent giddiness and vomiting. There was no ataxia, however, and the giddiness, as with others, was related to movements of the head. On the second day, he developed the transient nystagmus seen in many of these cases. This remitted in a week, but years later he succumbed to a classical attack of Bornholm disease, which also remitted in about a month. Again, culture of coxsackie B virus was positive from the stools.

Guillain-Barré Syndrome

M17

M17 was a fourteen-year-old boy, who was an only child. He and his father had suffered from a febrile flulike illness for three days prior to calling me in 1962. Upon examination, I was concerned that he had an ascending type of paresis and required hospitalization. It was arranged and he was admitted, but the paralysis was more severe the following day, and he required treatment on the respirator available at the time. He had a lumbar puncture and, though no cells were present in the CSF, there was a high protein content. An enterovirus was cultured from his stools, but we have no record of its precise grouping. He had a stormy time and still has some residual paresis, chiefly of his lower limbs.

Progressive Muscular Atrophy (PMA) (Aran-Duchenne Type)

F21

This woman was forty-two years old, and in 1980 had a rather severe viral illness. Her titers to Coxsackievirus rose as follows: B1, 1/8; B2, 1/128; B3, 1/128; B4, 1/32; B5, 1/32; B6, 1/8. The ELISA IgM and IgG tests were also positive. We did not culture the stools. The primary illness remitted, and for a few months she appeared to be recovering, save for weakness, etc. However, muscle wasting began to occur in the arms, legs, and intrinsic muscles and progressed without remission. She eventually became totally paralyzed, except (oddly) for her right thumb. I visited her regularly, and she was a wonderful patient, but sadly she died due to the usual paralytic respiratory effects of her illness and the resultant bronchopneumonia. Other workers have found enteroviral sequences in the spinal cords in other cases of motor neuron disease.

M18

This forty-six-year-old man was one of the first cases I saw when I was in private practice in 1939. This man, after a viral illness (which at the time caused interest in medical circles as poliomyelitis was around), began to show weakness of the intrinsic muscles of the hands and also developed fasciculations. This later spread centrally to affect the whole of the arms and legs. I took him to see Dr. Franklin Bicknell on Wimpole Street in London, as at that time he had an interest in alphatocopherol as a means of hindering the development of free oxygen radicals. However, this man's course was as unremitting as the previous case and he died from pulmonary complications after a long illness.

M19

This man was seen first in 1973 and is a good example of the sequelae of viral illness in a single individual in a family. His daughter had an evanescent viral illness from which she recovered. He also had an episode of severe abdominal pain and watery diarrhea. His coxsackie B group 4 titers rose to more than 1/512, and later he had a positive ELISA IgM. Within a month, he developed a myopericarditis, and months later, his serological titers were recorded as 1/1024 for coxsackie B group 4. This remitted, but he had a recurrence in 1978 and on this occasion had a viral pneumonitis; again his coxsackie B group 4 titers rose to 1/1024. He was seen by my partner and by the chest physician of the day, and they thought that he was developing stenosing alveolitis.

In 1980, he had a rather severe attack of vertigo and became somewhat unstable. After a careful examination I judged this to be cerebellar. In 1983, he developed the classic irritable bowel syndrome referred to earlier and also proctalgia, which was investigated, though no local cause was found. I considered it to be hypothalamically mediated. At the same time he developed a myelodysplastic syndrome with peripheral blast cells that were not characteristic of pernicious anemia. To complicate the picture, he began to have epileptiform attacks and over the next few years also developed evidence of central and peripheral motor neuron disease. Again, over the years, the disease progressed relentlessly, and as in the previous cases he became totally paralyzed. This, together with the stenosing alveolitis, resulted in his death in 1990. A summary of his syndromes would include Bornholm disease with myopericarditis, later pneumonitis and stenosing alveolitis, later still IBS and proctalgia, disequilibrium, dysplastic marrow syndrome, and finally progressive muscular atrophy motor neuron disease. This case is a sinister warning to our profession to look for a possible common etiogical cause for consequential illness.

F22

This child was born to parents, who were affected by coxsackie B at the time of conception. This was in 1973. The father died due to a coxsackie-induced cardiomyopathy shortly after the child was born. His history is in Chapter 2 as case M11, and also Chapter 4 as Family 01. Photographs of the child as a baby show the large mouth and flabby, fat arms (see Figure 3.2). The large mouth was also evident later in life.

The term amyotonia congenita seems to have been discarded but is the only appropriate term here, as the condition did progress, until as a fifteen-year-old she was tube fed and died in a hospital abroad. I owe gratitude to the hospital physicians who relayed continual up-to-date findings to me, including a chromosome analysis, which was normal. Apparently she had titers of 1/256 for coxsackie B group 2 and also 1/512 for group 4, but all other viral titers were negative. It was apparent from

FIGURE 3.2 Child Born to Parents Who Were Affected by Coxsackie B

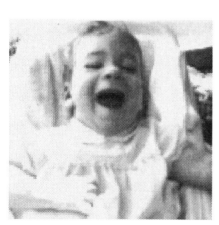
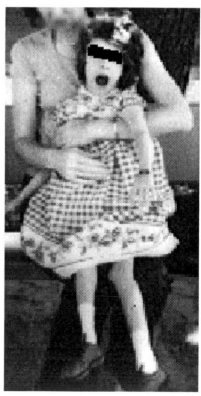

her presentation as a baby that she had suffered an intrapartum viral infection, and that these were the ongoing sequelae.

M20

This child is referred to in Chapter 7 also, but should be mentioned here as he was born to a mother who had severe Bornholm disease in the last trimester. Her titers of coxsackie B group were 1, 1/8; 2, 1/8; 3, 1/250; 4, 1/8; 5, 1/128; 6, 1/8. Her complement (CH50) fell to 46 and she had a positive ELISA IgM. The baby was delivered normally and was monitored carefully. At about fourteen weeks it was obvious he had some abnormal reflexes, and a CAT scan demonstrated severe but localized brain damage (see Figure 3.3). His physical functions are now quite good, and mentally he is quite bright. He has only a partially palsied right forearm. He recently passed his driving test but, unhappily, since then has had one epileptic fit. His titers as a baby to coxsackie B virus were as follows: 1, 1/8; 2, 1/256; 3, 1/8; 4, 1/256; 5, and 6, 1/8. His elder brother also was tested and his titers were identical to those of the mother. A later MRI scan demonstrates the extent of the lesion.

FIGURE 3.3 M20's Brain

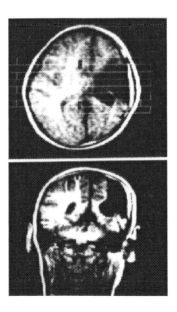

Multiple Sclerosis

Multiple Sclerosis may have an acute episode and remit entirely (a condition that could be termed pseudo or possible multiple sclerosis), or it might be subacute and pursue a relapsing course over years, or maybe, as in a few, be unremitting and relentless over years with a fatal ending. There is evidence for each of these stages in the series studied here. Moreover, it is perhaps sinister that there is serological and histological evidence for a viral etiology in most cases, whether of the remitting or progressive type. Examples are given, plus MRI images that are clearly positive in two cases that have proved to be MS. It is maybe significant that in both cases the serological picture was similar to that seen in the other listed syndromes.

It might also be significant that in the affective disorder of schizophrenia a similar pattern of acute or chronic sequential illness has been seen as in other disorders such as encephalitis lethargica, progressive supranuclear palsy, and subcortical dementia due to basal ganglia damage. That the common origin is related to Coxsackievirus infection appears likely (Peatfield, 1987). Some CNS disorders we have encountered are not due to viral infections and in my experience have occurred in cases of insidious TB infection and as a result of insecticide poisoning.

F23

One female child about five years of age presented with irrational temper tantrums and would not sit still for examination. She was taken to the beach, where she played with sand castles, and only exhibited her temper when her play was interrupted. The same evening she was brought to my surgery, cyanosed and in status epilepticus. I had to transport her to the hospital by car after giving her a Valium injection. Lumbar puncture defined the illness as tuberculous meningitis (TBM), and her mother was subsequently found to have a small active lung lesion. Both recovered.

M21

An elderly pensioner had been accused of micturating in telephone booths, which he thought were toilets. He had an ESR of 100 and signs of pulmonary disease as well as an acute type of dementia. The duly authorized officer (DAO) of the day refused to certify him as mentally ill and the following day the pensioner's body was recovered from the river. Postmortem examination showed an active TB lesion, as expected, together with signs of TBM.

M22

This man in his early forties presented with an ESR of 100 and a large loin abscess. It was drained in the hospital and the only report was that "no malignant cells were seen." Unhappily the abscess recurred, and on aspiration I found caseous fluid and Zeil-Neilson staining showed one TB bacillus. Investigations dragged on for about a year, and the diagnosis of TB was not accepted until he developed a typical psoas abscess. He was then given routine antitubercular treatment but developed a schizophrenic type of psychosis that required hospitalization for a while. He has gradually improved.

These three cases are mentioned lest the impression is given that only a virus can be cited as the causative agent. However, in the viral context the following cases occurred.

F24

F24 was a thirty-five-year-old patient who was seen in 1978. She had a typical onset of Bornholm disease. Her titers of coxsackie B group 4 were 1/512, and she had positive ELISA IgM and later IgG. Many years later she had a positive VP1 test. No other viral titer was significant. This progressed to a typical myocarditis, for which she had to be admitted to the hospital. After a stormy two years and gamma globulin infusions this resolved. She later developed weakness of her limbs and, as in the case of another young woman, she asked whether this was the onset of multiple sclerosis, as her aunt was said to have developed it. Both of these patients, in fact, developed brisk long-tract reflexes, had extensor Babinski reflexes, and lost their abdominal reflexes. However, in both cases the signs remitted and now, years later, they are well and free from symptoms. This raises the question once again as to the possibility of an acute form of MS that does in fact entirely remit.

F25

This woman had an illness identical to the previous case during the same years, except that she did not have myocarditis. However, she had all the signs and symptoms of MS and was investigated in a hospital, where her lumbar puncture and other findings were normal, with no conclusion forthcoming. Her coxsackie B titers of both groups 2 and 4 rose to 1/512, and she had a positive ELISA IgM and a positive VP1 when that test became available. She is still incapacitated and scores 20/25 on the ME Scoring Chart. She depends upon an electric wheelchair for locomotion and fits into the ME category. MRI imaging of her brain and spinal cord shows no evidence of MS, and the diagnosis is now ME. However, if a doctor who did not know the case could see her, I have no doubt the issue of MS would be raised again. Incidentally, it has been shown that ME also occurs in animals, and the dog belonging to this family developed diabetes and all the symptoms and signs of ME. The dog's blood has shown positive in a VP1 test.

F26

I first saw this thirty-six-year-old woman in 1987. She was sent to me as a possible ME case, but on examination she had all the CNS signs of MS. It is interesting that she only scored 3 on our ME scoring chart. However, the diagnosis of MS was refused at the time. In 1991, she was referred to me again, as she could only walk with the aid of arm crutches. On examination she had very brisk long-tract reflexes with mild unsustained clonus, absent abdominal reflexes and extensor plantar reflexes. On funduscopy she had temporal pallor of the optic discs suggestive of MS. On repeating her tests it was found that she had, as before, a titer suggesting past coxsackie B virus infection. In 1987 her ELISA IgM had been positive, and later she also had a positive IgG. This time, in 1991, a VP1 test was also done, which was highly positive and continues to be so. MRI imaging was performed and shows the typical lesions in the brain and spinal cord (as shown in Figure 3.4).

She has been treated with IgG infusions and has improved to the extent that she no longer needs any support for walking.

FIGURE 3.4. Typical Lesions in the Brain and Spinal Cord

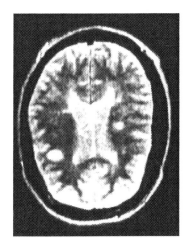 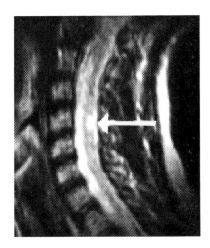

F27

This woman, who was born in 1960, was first ill in 1986 with a rather typical viral illness and intense radicular pain and quickly developed the signs and symptoms of a demyelination syndrome. Her sight was also affected. She could not drive her car, and reading was mostly impossible. She had an eightfold rise of titers of coxsackie B virus group 5 and later a rise to groups 2, 3, and 4. The ELISA IgM and IgG tests were also positive, and later her VP1 was positive. Later still, the acute stage remitted and she became fairly well. I delivered her children and they were normal. In 1989 and 1990 she relapsed and again had marked difficulty with her vision and once more had to give up driving. Her fundi showed the pallor of MS, chiefly the right fundus, but this also remitted. MRI imaging was undertaken, which showed diffuse lesions in the brain and spinal cord. Her MRI scan is almost identical to that shown for case F26.

These cases have been treated with gamma globulin therapy on a fairly intense and prolonged basis, and all have done well. The last case has remitted, is driving her car, and can read well.

MALIGNANCY OF THE CNS

It is not my purpose to go into details except to say that sixteen malignancies of the CNS have occurred in this study. They were mostly gliomas, with one astrocytoma. The ages ranged from forty to sixty years, but one was a young woman in her twenties. They all had serological evidence of enteroviral infection and a previous illness due to it. One man was tentatively diagnosed in 1989 or 1990. It could not be proven, but he later went into the terminal stages with a brain tumor and has died.

HYPOTHALAMIC AND BASAL GANGLIA-MEDIATED SYNDROMES

In this study, varying syndromes have been reported that probably result from neurological or neurohormonal effects of the hypothalamic nuclei. A brief resume of some of the considerations is as follows.

The corpus striatum is made up of the caudate and lenticular nuclei. It is the infracortical center for the regulation of extrapyramidal impulses. Lesions in this area produce disturbances of muscle tone together with involuntary movements but no true paralysis. The functions of the striatum are motor or efferent whereas those of the thalamus are afferent. The striatum receives its afferent impulses through the thalamus. Its fibers lead downward to the red nucleus and through it they innervate muscles on both sides of the body, but mainly the contralateral parts.

Thus, it is an accessory pathway with connections with the motor nuclei and the spinal cord via relays in the reticular formation. It is generally felt that the influence of the caudate nucleus inhibits and regulates movements initiated by the cerebral cortex. In cases of degeneration or atrophy of the corpus striatum, rigidity (and tremor independent of the rigidity) can occur and points to the lack of control by the caudate nucleus. There is a balance between the cortical efferent-stimulated movements and the striatal efferent-inhibiting effects.

Lesions of the caudate-neo-striatal system, which is inhibitory, can be followed by choreic or athetoid movements. Huntington's chorea, which is an extreme genetic example, gives a full-blown picture of what can arise if the inhibitory effects of the striatum are lost.

Some cases of dystonia musculorum deformans have been shown to follow encephalitis that was presumably of viral origin. While these are extreme examples, in this series the effects of assumed viral encephalitis have been shown to produce some of these symptoms and also include a Parkinson-like syndrome that has been reported in children.

Thus, the common link is this striatal system. We have evidence that it is affected from SPECT scans that show hypoperfusion. Figure 3.5 shows these relationships.

FIGURE 3.5. Midbrain Striatal System

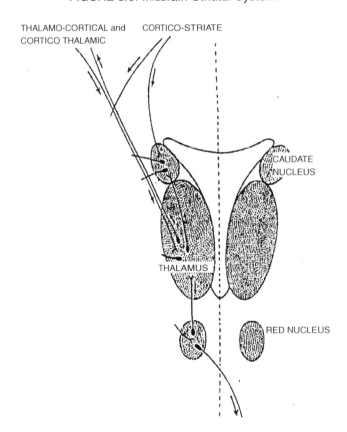

Case Studies

One case that illustrates the effects of virus on the basal ganglia will suffice.

M24

M24 was a fifteen-year-old boy who was brought in during 1994. He had taken ill in 1992 with violent abdominal pain, diarrhea and vomiting. Later his sleep pattern was reversed to owl 3 and his speech became almost inaudible. His limbs were so weak that he could not walk, and he could scarcely raise his arms. He was so grossly fatigued that he could hardly function. He developed serious photophobia and hyperacusis. On examination, I found a Parkinson-like picture with all the features of that condition (see Figure 3.6). When he attempted to elevate his arms, he had gross pronator signs. He was pallid and had a gross forward stoop that was quite apparent when he was seated. He lacked concentration but did not have anomia. As with a

FIGURE 3.6. SPECT Scan of M24

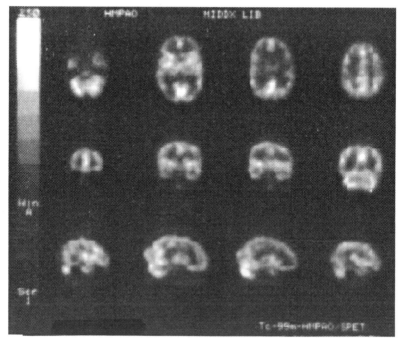

few others, his pupils were large and contracted mildly to light but not at all on accommodation. This reversal of the Argyll Robertson pupil has been referred to elsewhere and has been captured and retained on videotape. His grip was so poor that I gave consideration at the time to a diagnosis of myasthenia gravis, but eventually this was ruled out. He has been treated with Eldepryl, IgG, and choline mixture and, so far, has made a 50 percent recovery. His serial VP1 tests have been positive for persisting enterovirus.

His SPECT scan, performed recently, and the graph is as shown in Figure 3.7. The graph demonstrates poor definition of the caudate nuclei on both sides, particularly of the right hemisphere, and also hypoperfusion to the brain stem/hypothalamus.

FIGURE 3.7. Graphical Representation of M24

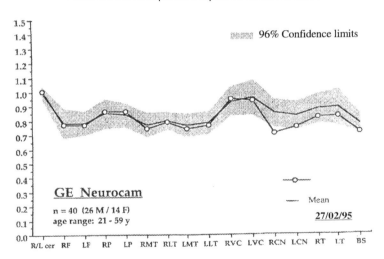

Dr. D. C. Costa, who performed this scan, gave an excellent lecture, "Single Photon Emission Tomography (SPET) in ME Patients" at the Research Workshop of the Newcastle Research Group in 1995. The objective was "To investigate the brain perfusion of patients with ME/CFS in comparison with normal volunteers, patients with depression to test the hypothesis that brainstem hypoperfusion is a characteristic of patients with ME/CFS and is not present in patients with depression" (Costa, 1995). His results and conclusions were presented as follows:

Results—The quantitative analysis of the brain perfusion SPET studies demonstrated that ME/CFS patients showed generalised reduction (statistically significant) of the brain perfusion in the majority of the brain regions (frontal, parietal, temporal lobes, thalamus and caudate nucleus in both hemispheres, as well as the brainstem) compared to normal controls. The more marked and highly statistically significant (p < 0.0001 using ANOVA) differences were found in the brainstem, frontal lobes and right caudate nucleus. Patients with major depression had reduced brain perfusion in the frontal, parietal and right temporal lobes, as well as the right caudate nucleus, statistically significant at the 0.0001 level using ANOVA with Bonferroni correction for multiple comparisons. However, the brainstem of patients with major depression was within normal limits. The ten patients with epilepsy showed normal perfusion ratios to the brainstem. Table 3.2 below shows the brainstem perfusion ratios for normals, ME/CFS, depressed and epileptic patients.

TABLE 3.2. Brainstem Perfusion Ratios

	Normal	ME/CFS	Depression	Epilepsy
No.	40	67	20	10
Mean BS	0.795	0.734	0.773	0.811
1 SD	0.032	0.047	0.030	0.067
p (vs. Normal)	—	<0.0001	ns	ns
p (vs. Depression)	ns	= 0.0004	—	ns

Figure 3.8 demonstrates the distribution of perfusion ratios obtained on a patient with typical ME/CFS (A) and on a patient with major depression (B) compared with the data from the normal database (mean ±2 SD).

Conclusions—Our data indicate that brain perfusion in ME/CFS is lower than normal and more interestingly that brainstem perfusion is significantly lower than in patients with major depression and appears to be characteristic of ME/CFS patients. In addition, brainstem hypoperfusion may be due to an abnormality with organic substrate, at least at the biochemical or metabolic level. Furthermore, this objective test of brain perfusion with SPET may be used to assess response to therapy, playing an important role in the investigation of drug efficacy in the treatment of ME/CFS patients.

FIGURE 3.8. Distribution of Perfusion Ratios Obtained on a Patient with Typical ME/CFS (A) and on a Patient with Major Depression (B) Compared with the Data from the Normal Database (Mean ±2 SD)

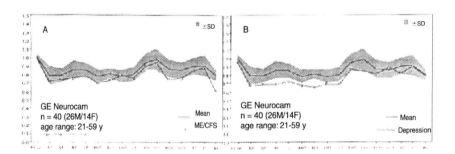

I am very grateful to Dr. Costa for releasing the results of this work, some of which relate to patients that I referred, and it will be seen that these scans are identical with the one shown for case M24. The benefits of these scans are now becoming more evident and reflect the increase in their use. A further example indicates the hypoperfusion of basal ganglia (see Figure 3.9). The MRI in this case was normal, thus illustrating that the abnormality was due not to anatomical but to a physiological abnormality. Whether this abnormality can be corroborated by the positive buspirone tests is worthy of consideration. The basic reason for this hypoperfusion is now a challenge for further research.

As epilepsy does occur as an isolated entity in some cases, it also can be shown that abnormal EEGs occur in a considerable proportion of cases of postviral encephalitis. This is illustrated in the following case report.

F28

Patient F24 had a coxsackie B group 4 infection in 1984 and, as usual, the antibody titers and IgM, as well as VP1 tests later, were all

FIGURE 3.9. MRI Indicating Hypoperfusion of Basal Ganglia

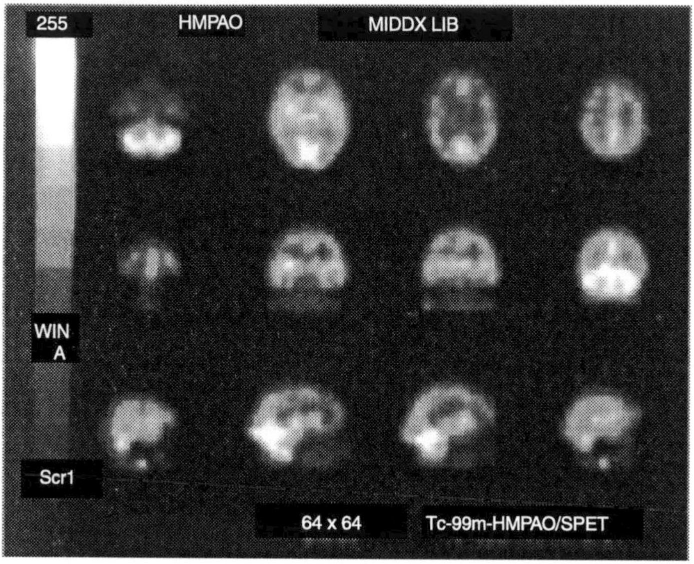

highly positive. Two months after the illness, she developed a severe intellectual disability and stated that "Things were not registering with me, I experience strange sensations and feel my body is there but I am not. I feel as if I was far away, my speech was slurred and slow and I could not do any calculations." She also complained of vague pains in the head, anomia, and an inability to read. This was followed by clusters of abnormal sensations which she described as "Something closing in my head, and at times, a sensation of brightness which seemed to tunnel in." She felt as though at times she was losing consciousness but was still aware of her surroundings, though her movements were shaky and slow. She noticed that reading was almost impossible, and any attempt to read resulted in "feeling the same sensations, with tremor, letters going out of focus, and something like a flickering light appearing." She had no other outward effects and did not lose consciousness but was unable to continue reading or to understand the text.

An early CAT brain scan was normal, but an EEG at the time was abnormal. Since then, an MRI scan was also normal, but a PET scan showed an area of relatively increased tracer accumulation lying in the left hemisphere in the lower parietal lobe in the region of the insular. The measured regions of interest in this site differed from the contralateral; the differences varied from 7 percent to 13 percent. This site was the same focal area as on an earlier scan and corresponded to the EEG abnormal recording localized to the left temporal region and showed a focal increased tracer accumulation corresponding to the active seizure source.

We finally performed a long video EEG recording (as shown in Figure 3.10) during alert stages and during reading. This showed a posterior rhythm in the distribution of alpha, which is fast at around 15 Hertz. This was symmetrical and was attenuated when she opened her eyes. There were frequent focal abnormalities consisting of runs of theta waves or sharp and slow waves localized around the left anterior temporal electrode. Independent of this, there were similar, but less frequent abnormalities, around the right anterior temporal electrode.

FIGURE 3.10. F28's EEG Recording During Alert Stages and Reading

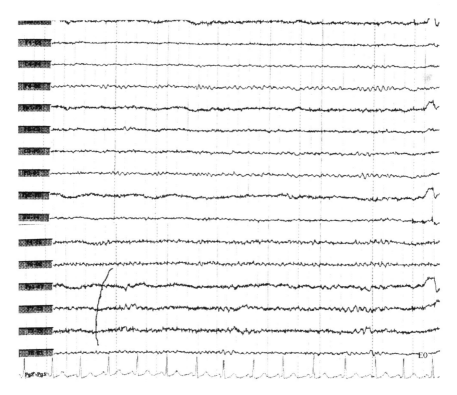

Intermittent photic stimulation evoked a marked response and, on one occasion, a brief abortive burst on both sides. These consisted of small larval spikes. During long periods of reading, she was unable to understand what she was reading, but this was not associated with EEG changes though she complained of a dizzy head, her eyes going out of focus, and a feeling of body vibration. It was felt that there was no objective EEG evidence of actual reading-induced seizures, but rather that the consistent EEG changes were evidence of functional abnormalities which themselves were expressed by her alexia.

F29

Another case was referred to me from one of my colleagues. The woman had suffered a viral illness, as evidenced by her high titers. She scored 19/25 on our ME Scoring Chart. She had accentuated upper and lower limb reflexes and severe muscular jitter, with softened "infarcted" areas in both thigh and calf muscles. Her eyes and retinal fundi were normal, and her ESR was 10 mm in one hour. Her GE Neurocam is shown in Figure 3.11 and is typical of the pattern seen in these cases.

FIGURE 3.11. F29's GE Neurocam

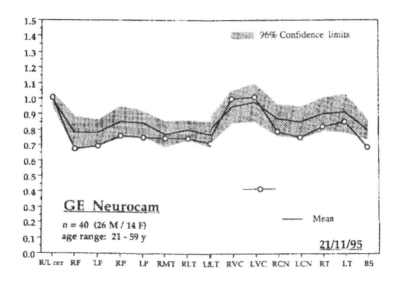

F30

The complexity of virus-mediated illness is also well demonstrated in this case. Five years prior to being seen she had experienced an episode of severe abdominal pain that at first was thought to come from her gallbladder, then perhaps her ovaries, and later her stomach. Various X rays were performed but did not confirm these diagnoses. Some time later, she wakened one morning and found she had lost the sight in her right eye and had an episode of vision defect in her left eye that was not nearly so severe. She was investigated for the possibility of MS, but the lumbar puncture was normal. She complained of many symptoms that did not fit into the diagnosis of MS, and general examination did not confirm this diagnosis. However, her right fundus was extremely pale while her left fundus was normal.

She had joined an MS support group but felt she did not have the symptoms that she observed in the other members and thus sought further help. On examination, she scored 18/25 on the ME Score Chart and thus had many of the symptoms associated with this condition. Her serology showed a rise in coxsackie B group titers as follows: 1, 1/8; 2, 1/128; 3, 1/32; 4, 1/32; 5, 1/512; 6, 1/8. Polio virus titers were: 1, 1/32; 2, 1/256; 3, 1/32. Her VP1 test was positive.

The clinical presentation was different from many others, and the possibility of subacute myelo-optico-neuropathy arose. Further blood was taken and the sera separated, and a colleague who worked in this viral field kindly took the sample to the United States for testing for the Inoue-Melnic virus, for which it was positive. Later MRI scanning was performed, which did not show any of the stigma of MS.

She has also had treatment with IgG intramuscular infusions and the choline mixture. Her progress has been very satisfactory. This case is presented to show the unusual considerations that may arise in the viral field of pathology.

MYALGIC ENCEPHALOMYELITIS

Nowhere is a variety of systemic symptoms seen more often than in myalgic encephalomyelitis. While it is a defined entity, other organ pathology is not infrequent and can obscure the picture. In this series about 25 percent also developed other antibodies, and antithyroid antibodies occurred in about 20 percent of cases. A lecture given at Cambridge in 1990 summarizes this syndrome (Nightingale Research Foundation, 1991).

Much has been written on the subject. It has been treated as a myth, or as a single entity that was then claimed by some to be psychiatric or by others to be organic in origin. In the first group, labels were applied ranging from depression to hysteria while in the second, valid observation as well as vague hypotheses are still the order of the day. This merely illustrates the limitations of the medical mind in fully explaining the fundamental pathology of all illness.

The observations in the following sections are the result of continuous follow-up and analysis of sequential illness in patients varying in situation and time over a period of forty years.

Prevalence and Clinical Diagnosis

As with poliomyelitis, surveys have shown ME to be epidemic, endemic, and also sporadic. It may follow an acute viral illness such as Bornholm disease, pericarditis, labyrinthitis, or meningoencephalitis. A more vague flulike illness with chest or bowel disturbance may be the harbinger of a more insidious onset. Apparent malaise not only fails to end but becomes more defined, developing symptoms such as anomia or severe concentration difficulty in a previously highly accomplished person who now cannot recall a paragraph even after reading it several times. Muscle power may not appear to be affected, but if examined carefully, softened and very tender areas may be demonstrated. Muscle jitter is a feature in 25 percent of these cases. This can be shown by seating the patient on the examination table and asking him or her to raise and lower the lower leg, whereby the jitter is easily seen. Concomitant myocardial or endocrine gland dysfunction also occurs, but if these resolve, the physician may be very frustrated to find that the patient is still ill. The graphs in Figure 3.12 show relative prevalence, and it is apparent that females do not predominate as some have thought, given the overall CNS sequelae to viral illness. Since these graphs were developed, the absolute number of cases being considered has risen, but the percentages have remained unchanged.

FIGURE 3.12. Analysis of Pure ME and CNS Pathology of Patients by Sex

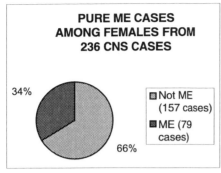

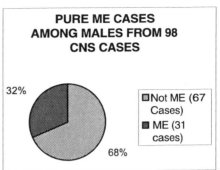

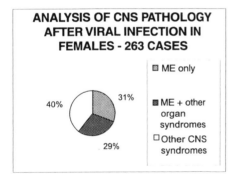

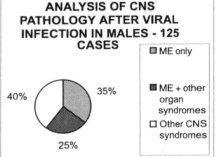

Quantification of Symptoms in Myalgic Encephalomyelitis

I devised the scoring chart shown in Table 3.3 in the early 1960s to summarize the symptoms that were recorded by patients in their own written histories of this illness. There were approximately 300 such written histories, and the symptoms that form the basis of this chart occurred in 80 percent of the cases.

If the patient qualifies for the diagnosis for each question, then the score indicated in the third column is recorded in the fourth column. The sum of the values in this fourth column then represents the patient's overall score. Answering these questions, therefore, yields a global view of the symptoms that occur in ME. An overall score of

TABLE 3.3. Myalgic Encephalitis Scoring Chart

1.	Has there ever been any evidence, either illness or titer, of past viral infection?	1
2.	FATIGUE	
(a)	Are you less than 33 percent efficient per full day (including hobbies after work, etc.)	2
(b)	Do you need a period of bed or settee rest:	
	- during each day?	3
or	- on 2 or 3 days per week?	2
3.	Have you excessive fatigue after work effort?	2
4.	Do you have nocturnal sweats or cold feelings?	2
5.	EVIDENCE OF DISTURBED MENTAL ACTIVITY	
(a)	Do you have difficulty finding the correct words?	1
(b)	Can you write a long letter without your handwriting ability deteriorating?	1
(c)	Do you tire if you have to talk for long?	1
6.	FAINT ATTACKS (VASOMOTOR CNS INSTABILITY)	
(a)	Do you tend to have faint attacks:	
	- and lose consciousness?	3
or	- without loss of consciousness but have to sit or lie down?	2
7.	Do you feel fatigued upon waking?	1
8.	Can you stand a lot of "chatter" (Hyperacusis)?	1
9.	Do you have cold or numb feelings in your extremities or face?	2
10.	Is your gait consistent with your age or is it that of a person much older or unsteady?	1
	TOTAL	

fifteen or more is highly suggestive of the condition and can be broken down into four sections:

1. *Fatigue.* This can be either central fatigue or muscle fatigue. Central fatigue is probed in question 7 while peripheral fatigue is indicated by questions 3 and 10. The resulting combination would be suggested by question 2 (a) and (b). Muscle fatigue is known to be related to an excess of lactic acid after work effort. In this condition, however, excessive activity is usually reflected the following day, and it may take days for the patient to recover.

2. *Mental Activity.* Question 5(a) indicates anomia, which is a very well recognized symptom in this condition, while question 5(b) reflects the motor fatigue involved in transposing verbal to written language. This may indicate the involvement of supra- and infrasensorial mechanisms within the brain and may also be evidenced by a positive response to question 5(c).

3. *CNS Instability.* This is seen in varying degrees of severity in 80 percent of the cases, hence the two grades of response to question 6(a). The test for the former is performed by placing the patient prone on the examination couch and performing serial ECGs and carefully monitoring blood pressure. The backrest is then raised to 45° and blood pressure recorded at two-minute intervals. If any change in heart rate is detected, then further ECGs are performed. After five minutes the patient is asked to stand upright, and further blood pressures are recorded. In only 10 percent of cases is there a significant change in heart rate, but changes in blood pressure as indicated usually occur. In the supine position, the blood pressure normally is quite low but in the 45° position often rises by 50 mm systolic and 20 mm diastolic. When the patient assumes the erect position it again falls to levels either equal to or below those recorded for the supine position. Only in the small minority of cases with a concomitant bradycardia did a collapse occur, but, as indicated, many of the other patients felt weak and had to sit down.

Question 8 again alludes to the central fatigue in which the patient has a limited ability to absorb information. On occasion, certain tones become extremely painful, constituting the "tensor tympani" syndrome.

Question 9 relates to vasomotor instability reflected in temperature or sensory changes, which again may reflect abnormal reception in the hypothalamic nuclei.

4. *Overall Result.* Finally, question 10 is obviously the result of a conglomeration of the other symptoms.

The Differential Diagnosis of Myalgic Encephalomyelitis

Obviously the history obtained is of first importance. In the cases so far, it is striking how consistent the symptoms are that characterize this condition. Moreover, when the cases are studied in retrospect, the following fact emerges. Approximately 7,000 cases of viral illness over four decades have been listed and broken down into five groups. The first contained over 5,000 cases who had had quite a severe illness but recovered without sequelae within six months. However, just under 20 percent of this group did have a recurrence of enteroviral origin at a future date but not always with the same syndrome, e.g., one case had Bornholm disease and the second attack was viral meningitis. These were chiefly enteroviral cases, and it is interesting that no one in Group 1 progressed to postviral illness, be it ME or another syndrome. However, of all 7,000 cases, 1,670 did have postviral syndromes, some from the original attack and some who had a recurrent illness (Group 2).

It is of interest to note that some of the initial illnesses appeared to clear completely (e.g., meningitis or Bornholm disease), while others (e.g., pericarditis, myocarditis, nephritis, etc.), could remit or pursue a more chronic course. A lifelong syndrome (e.g., diabetes) might ensue in a small minority. Yet again, in a small minority with acute onset there are those who do not make a recovery and develop ME. The difficulty of diagnosis is compounded by the fact that in many cases, none of the severe initial syndromes may have presented. In fact it might be assumed that a severe, acute illness provoked a host response with complete remission, while a subacute illness did not. However, there is an overlap, and as usual it is probably too facile to be dogmatic.

Thus, for the purpose of differential diagnosis two main conditions should be considered, namely, the pathogenic agent and the organ affected. The host response should also be seen as a third condition that vitally affects these two factors. Considered separately in the context of the condition studied here, this can be summarized as follows.

Pathogenic Agent

Pathogenic agents may be organic or inorganic. In the present context most organic pathogens are viral, but, as shown later, this is not exclusive of other agents. Most of the inorganic agents are varying chemical toxins, and of these the insecticides used on farms for crops or animals, or in the home for insects on plants and occasionally for lice on children or pets, together with wood preservatives used in the home or at work, are the most common in the United Kingdom. This is not exclusive and could be extended to the ingestion of toxins on food or in water, etc. We have recorded such cases, which have caused profound paresis in some cases and in others subclinical weakness that could be classified as ME.

Organs Affected

It is obvious that either organic or inorganic toxins may have an effect on varying organs and thus give rise to varying syndromes described under various titles. This depends not only on the toxin but also on the host.

Host Response

Host response is a crucial consideration relating to the previous considerations. In the case of organisms, be they virus or others, it can be shown that the host response may determine the degree as well as the site of infection. Some patients may be immune to certain organisms while others may be susceptible. The degree of immunity may vary over months or years and also be suppressed by varying factors (e.g., toxins), which then act as cofactors. While we are aware of this, other host factors that appear to influence organ susceptibility are not so well understood. It is interesting that antibodies may be general and circulating in serum or they may be purely local.

I showed this thirty years ago while investigating cases of infertility, where sperm subjected to only one minute of contact with cervical mucin died, but would survive a whole night in the female's serum. When a viral infection occurs in a family, one member may have cardiac and another CNS involvement, while the others remain free of illness. Thus a single agent may be responsible for differing syndromes. This may be explained by "local cell surface" acting antibodies with specific organ-protective qualities, but these antibodies also can vary over the years. Taking this into account, the differential diagnosis should not be taken to imply a different etiology. Another corollary is that identical causes, with differing syndromes, would respond to the same treatment. However, bearing this in mind, it is also important to see that multiorgan involvement may occur due to infection; also, the involvement of one organ may have effects on other organs. This is well demonstrated in the hypothalamic region, which has a wide supervisory role, operated via neuronal and humeral mechanisms. Examples of these mechanisms can be seen more centrally in pituitary regulation, with its further effects from the thyroid, adrenals, etc. to the apparently more distant regulation of bowel motility.

These factors make an exclusive title for an illness difficult. In diabetes there is not just pancreatic involvement, because the Kimmelstiel-Wilson syndrome, which involves multiorgan sequelae, shows how diffuse the effects may be. Also in anterior poliomyelitis other neurological involvement takes place apart from that in the motor system. Autonomic disturbance is perhaps the most frequent, and hyper- or hypohidrosis, systemic hypertension, and gastric hypomotility or atony with constipation, as well as sensory loss due to the posterior roots of the cord being affected, have all been recorded (Plum, 1956). In my series, cerebellar ataxia, papilloedema due to increased intracranial pressure, and Reye's syndrome have also occurred in the acute infective stage of viral illness, and these conditions were also reported by Curnen and colleagues (1961) and Brunberg and colleagues. The progression from the acute to the more chronic stage in all these diseases may not follow an orderly pattern either in time or organ location, which may be diffuse, and this is reflected in the ME syndrome.

We can briefly consider some of the factors involved in virus-host interchange. Viruses are intracellular obligate parasites, and the host mechanism has to recognize this if it is to deal effectively with the virus. The T cell population only recognizes antigen when it is displayed on cell membranes along with a cell marker. These markers belong to the major histocompatibility group (MHC). The T cells, if thus primed to the viral antigen, recognize and bind to it and the MHC molecule and commence to produce interferons (IFNs). Antibodies, complement, and polymorphonuclear leukocyte deal with circulating extracellular infection, while T cells, IFNs, macrophages, and NK cells deal with intracellular infection—in this case viral. This mechanism can be thwarted by so-called antigenic shift or drift. In the first, there is movement of genomic material, while in the second, there is a swapping of genetic material from reservoirs of different viruses. This could explain the way in which one infection reactivates a latent strain.

However, both local and systemic antibodies attempt to block the replication and spread of viruses, either circulating or being shed from a cell that has been infected and killed. IgG is the most prevalent antibody of the immunoglobulin system and is a potent opsonizing agent. The complement system of serum proteins is activated by IgM and later by IgG. They opsonize target cells for the phagocytes, which are then bound by IgM or IgG, and this is the classical pathway. Cells synthesize interferon when infected by virus; it is secreted into extracellular fluid and binds to adjacent cells. Interferon-alpha is derived from lymphocytes and interferon-beta from fibroblasts and other cell types. The IFNs act on certain cell genes that either catalyse or retard factors responsible for protein synthesis, which in turn reduces mRNA translation, while another factor results in the degradation of host and viral mRNA. The total result is to establish a sort of cordon of uninfectable cells around the virus. Thus, viral replication is inhibited. In mice if interferon is inactivated by an antiserum, they succumb to a small viral dose. IFNs have at least three roles—to kill virus, to inhibit host cell division, and to modulate the activity of NK cells.

In ME, as with certain other viral illness, T cell dysfunction occurs, and Hamblin showed an increase in suppressor activity with T cell suppression of in vitro synthesis by normal B cells. Also, Caligiuri (1987) found 73 percent of ME cases had a decrease in the number of NK cells, and the T3 negative subset was reduced in 50 percent. This is interesting in the light of the foregoing remarks, and CD4 T cells migrate from blood to tissues in virus-induced disease as viruses are intracellular obligate parasites. The persistent viral infection cycle is complex.

There may be a primary acute illness that would qualify for a definition, or it may be followed by a series of other symptoms that would require further definition. In some initial infections the primary stage may not be evident, including diseases as diverse as TB and even AIDS, among many others. All of this is true of ME. Thus a search for the origin may not be helpful and the continuing multiorgan effects may be confusing. Investigations for the continuing reason for this are a challenge. In considering these problems, the differential diagnosis of the primary illness is obviously important, and in my series some of the final diagnoses arrived at are discussed here.

Acute illness may be as follows: Bornholm disease; viral meningitis or encephalitis; labyrinthitis; cerebellar syndrome; hand-foot-and-mouth disease; GI syndromes; pancreatitis; viral pneumonitis; spinal radiculopathies; nonspecific influenza-type febrile illness. In considering the differential diagnosis, the following section is a brief and incomplete survey of variables.

Acute Presentations

- Bornholm disease, which may mimic gallstone or renal colic, torsion of bowel and pleurisy, or even myocardial infarction.
- Meningitis and encephalitis, which may be bacterial.
- Labyrinthitis is viral in most cases, but may mimic a basilar artery insufficiency syndrome.
- Cerebellar syndrome may again mimic a vascular-mediated syndrome.
- Hand-foot-and-mouth disease, with or without iritis, is usually viral, but erythema chronicum migrans (ECM) must be kept in mind as Lyme disease can closely mimic ME. *Ixodes dammini,* I have been told, exist in deer as near my area as Sherwood Forest. I have had one case.
- G.I. syndromes, e.g., gastroenteritis and also pancreatitis, may also be bacterial, toxic, or viral. Radiculopathies also occur and may have varied etiologies, but a viral cause should always be considered.
- Flulike illnesses may have varied and obscure causes. Serological titers often are not performed, although it may well be wise to do so for future reference, in case chronic sequelae occur.

Chronic Sequelae

The more challenging task involves chronic sequelae, which is particularly true in ME as the effects may be neurological, hormonal, autoimmune, or myalgic in varying degrees, and the latter may involve the myocardium. All of these may be discrete but also may occur as an additive in ME, which of course tends to cause problems. Moreover, the difficulty lies in the fact that the pathogenesis of the acute stage might not have been accurately defined. Because of my interest, serological titers were usually performed on more than one occasion in those presenting with a well-defined illness as shown in the previous list, but some patients with a flulike illness did not present until secondary effects developed. In these, the definitive titers may have fallen and culture was often negative, but the VP1 test developed by Professor Mowbray has proved of considerable value for suggesting ongoing enteroviral infection.

Conditions considered in this work, which again are not exclusive:

- Brucellosis—This may be difficult to define, and only one was proven in this series. However, it can produce all the acute and chronic symptoms alluded to in this work. In the CNS, diverse spinal and cerebral syndromes occur, sometimes with paranoid delusions. Endocarditis may cause emboli with remote effects. As with toxins, this should be considered in those who work with animals. However, the ESR is high, and lesions may develop that mimic sarcoidosis. The ELISA IgM in the acute stage or IgG in the chronic stage should be assayed.
- Lyme disease—As with brucellosis, it is difficult to prove in the chronic stage, and I have only seen one, which was considered but never proven. Lyme disease causes ECM skin lesions in the acute stage, which may be confused with hand-foot-and-mouth (HFM) disease. In the later stage neurological, cardiac, and arthritic conditions may follow, as with viruses. Lyme disease, however, is due to a spirochete transmitted by ixodid ticks.
- Tuberculosis—One was referred as ME but had a very high ESR, which is most unusual in ME. TB may have an obscure location, as was the case here, which was eventually shown to be renal.
- Carcinomas—Again, they usually have a high ESR. This is dealt with in another context in Chapter 8 and may be primary or sequential.
- Endocrine—This is dealt with in Chapter 5, but thyroid antibodies as well as diabetes can develop in these patients and be a complication in the ME syndrome.
- CVS—Pericarditis, perimyocarditis, and myocarditis have all been noted in this series as discrete or additive. The additive cases still manifest the symptoms of ME after the cardiac condition resolves.
- CNS—A list of other syndromes that have followed well-documented viral illness has been listed, but most, in my experience, can be excluded by careful examination, using MRI scans, etc.

- Auto-immune—This is a difficult area, and autoimmune sequelae are well recognized following viral infection. However, they should be differentiated clinically as a separate entity or as an additive factor in ME.
- Toxins—A small number have been seen and serologically proven. They can give rise to serious illness and should be borne in mind. They do have a depressive effect on bone marrow, which also occurs with viral infections. Jacobson and colleagues published the results of a good study in 1987. In these cases the serum folate was low, below 3 μg/L, which is the lower limit of normal. They reported that in half to three-quarters of all such patients, an unexpectedly low serum folate was found. In twenty-nine patients it was as low as 1.6 μg/L. Patients with normal values had on average 5.8 μg/L. Folate is required for hemopoiesis and for the conversion of uridylate to thymidylate of DNA and for all other cells and tissues. It is necessary for the synthesis of purine rings and of RNA and proteins. All infection causes a bimodal response of the immune system in cellular multiplication and synthesis of immunoglobulins, both of which are folate dependent. Repair in pulmonary and skin lesions makes demands on folates also.

  A high incidence of folate deficiency was found in those who had viral skin rashes. Also, Behan and colleagues (1985) noted this folate lack in cases of ME. However, thirty or more years ago I noted the association between folate levels and fetal abnormality, particularly in tissues deriving from ectoderm. Not infrequently, this was also linked with a viral infection at or just before the time of conception. It is also relevant that insecticides have been incriminated in fetal abnormality. The question then arises as to whether virus or toxin lowers the folate to danger levels, or whether a low folate level allows the body to be susceptible to infection. I suspect the former, but it still begs the question—Is it the virus or the low folate that actually mediates the neonatal pathology or adult illness?

The question is sometimes asked, "Do women with ME have an increased risk of bearing children with an abnormality?" The simplistic answer is "No." However, I did a study in a group of women of childbearing age (seventeen to thirty-seven years) who had a viral illness with at least an eightfold rise in Coxsackievirus titer and had become pregnant or had developed the illness during the last trimester. In that study, 68.2 percent had normal children, but there was a rather high number, 31.8 percent, which were abnormal. Broken down, the abnormal cases included: two aborted (3.0 percent); six stillbirths (9.1 percent); eleven fetal abnormalities (16.7 percent); and two babies who died from cardiac complications (3.0 percent). However, I emphasize that this is not related to ME but does relate to the pathogenicity of the enteroviral group of viruses.

The important consideration, however, is that the syndromes outlined may all cause chronic illness, and some may actually coexist with ME and have the same etiology, while others may mimic the condition. A very careful history written by the patient, which both saves time and is much more reliable than question and answer (which may be biased), should, in most cases, define the issue. The exercise can alert us to the possibility of occult infection in conditions that may cause chronic malaise. The persistence of spirochetes and viruses should by now be well recognized, but the investigatory proceedings needed in some cases, in my opinion, require more intensive laboratory investigations.

It may be helpful to review the "response to stress" and see the interplay of neurological and hormonal activity, which can be seen as an "efferent" response by the host. By the same token, there is an "afferent" result from the response of the immune system. This integrated function determines the whole pathological scenario, felt by the patient and perhaps perceived by the medical investigator, but this depends upon signs, which are often less obvious than symptoms.

Disturbance of Hypothalmic Function in Patients with ME

Evidence has been presented showing a change in the distribution of hypothalamic blood flow in association with CFS/ME (Bakheit et al., 1992). It has been claimed that the subset of CFS/ME associated with evidence of persistent viral infection shows some evidence of disturbed hypothalamic function. Bakheit and colleagues (1992) described the clinical features of CFS/ME and listed objective findings that distinguished the organic as opposed to the functional parts of the malady. In addition to biochemical, histological, viral, and electro-myographic parameters, they grouped several systemic features that suggest disturbance of hypothalamic function.

The anxiolytic drug buspirone, one of the azopyrones, stimulates the release of prolactin by acting on the 5-HT receptors. The bus-pirone-prolactin response was studied in a subgroup of patients with CFS/ME and evidence of persistent enteroviral infection, as shown by the repeated detection of the group-specific protein of enteroviruses, VP1, in the blood (Bakheit et al., 1992). Family controls who were asymptomatic were studied at the same time. In addition to the re-sponse to buspirone, diurnal variations in cortisol and prolactin levels were studied. It was found that patients with CFS/ME had much greater rises in prolactin levels one hour after buspirone compared to controls. Cortisol level were elevated in the patients, but the rise was not significantly different between the two groups. There was a significant association between the pattern of sleep disturbance known as the owl syndrome and the ratio of pre- and post-buspirone prolactin levels.

Pilot studies I undertook have shown that buspirone stimulates prolactin release to a significantly greater degree in CFS/ME patients compared to controls or patients with primary depression. These studies pointed to the buspirone test as a means of localizing some features of CFS/ME to a disturbance of the hypothalamus. To sub-stantiate this possibility, the test was performed in a larger controlled series of cases, and the results were correlated with the severity of pa-tient's illness. Since Demitrack and colleagues (1991) produced some evidence for changing cortisol levels in CFS/ME, it seemed worthwhile to study the diurnal release of both cortisol and prolactin, in addition to the buspirone-stimulation test.

Methods

Patient selection. Five males and twenty-five females were stud-ied, all with an extended history of muscle fatigue associated with cognitive disorders. The fatigue syndrome was assessed by a general questionnaire produced and validated by the Newcastle Research Group over several decades. These patients also fulfilled the criteria set out in the CDC and Oxford studies for CFS/ME. (The NRG questionnaire is known and used in Britain.) Patients fulfilling the criteria for CFS/ME, with other systemic disease excluded as a cause, were subjected to a study of VP1 protein in the serum, on one or more occasions, to identify the group with persistent enteroviral infection. Twenty-five of those with a positive VP1 test, that is, of those with values for binding of the monoclonal antibody more than two standard deviations above those of normal controls, were used in this study. The disturbance of sleep pattern (the owl syndrome) was graded as follows:

Grade	Sleep Pattern
0	Normal sleep pattern.
1	Remain awake until 2 a.m.
2	Remain awake until 4 a.m.
3	Remain awake until 6 a.m. (This group shows a complete reversal of sleep pattern, thus turning night into day.)

Family members were used as controls in this study, so it was important to ensure that they were normal. They all had normal profiles when examined, and their symptoms were investigated using the same questionnaires as their relatives who had CFS/ME.

Many of the patients selected did have indirect evidence of potential hypothalamic dysregulation including hyperphagia and obesity, feelings of inappropriate heat and cold in their extremities, and, in the females, changes in the menstrual cycle. These last symptoms may be associated with prolactin-induced inhibition of LH-RH secretion. The mean ages of the female and male subjects were thirty-eight years (fifteen to forty-eight) and thirty-eight years (thirty to sixty) respectively. None had taken any drug during the previous six weeks. The women were all tested during the luteal phase of the menstrual cycle.

In the family controls, some were blood relatives and some were not (e.g., sister-in-law). Three proved to be of exceptional interest because they had adjusted their sleep patterns to nurse their ill daughters who had grade 3 owl syndrome; thus they worked through the night and slept during the day. This was reflected in their prolactin responses, which were among the highest of the controls.

Buspirone Stimulation Studies

Each patient and his or her respective family control were tested together. Blood was collected by venipuncture from both patient and control as close to 10 p.m. as possible and stored at 4°C overnight. Fasting blood samples were taken the following morning at 9 a.m. Both study subjects were then given 50 mg of buspirone orally, and they continued to fast until the third blood sample was taken one hour later. Bakheit and colleagues (1992) had used 60 mg, but in this series only 50 mg were used and produced satisfactory results. The specimens were taken immediately to the Biochemistry Department of the Queen Elizabeth Hospital for analysis. Plasma prolactin levels were measured at the Abbott Laboratories, Maidenhead, and cortisol levels were measured by radioimmunoassay (Becton-Dickinson, Oxford). A diurnal ratio was calculated as the evening/morning values and the stimulation ratio as the value after/before buspirone.

Statistical Analysis

Since the data in all groups proved to be positively skewed with a few outlying points, the nonparametric Mann-Whitney U-test was used. The relationship between the owl syndrome grade and the stimulation ratio was assessed by the Spearman rank correlation test.

Results

Cortisol. Patients and controls did not differ in the basal levels of cortisol, although diurnal variation was evident in both. In response to buspirone, the patients attained a higher concentration than the controls, significant at the $p < 0.05$ level, but there was no difference in the stimulation ratio produced by buspirone ($p = 0.084$) (See Figure 3.13).

Prolactin. The prolactin responses to buspirone are shown in Figure 3.14. The levels of prolactin did not differ between patients and controls in their evening or morning samples. With the numbers tested, the diurnal variation did not attain statistical significance. Both groups responded significantly to the ingestion of buspirone, but the patients showed a much greater rise than the controls. The mean ratio for the patients was more than three times that of their familial controls ($p < 0.001$).

FIGURE 3.13. Cortisol (nmol/L) Responses in CFS/ME Patients

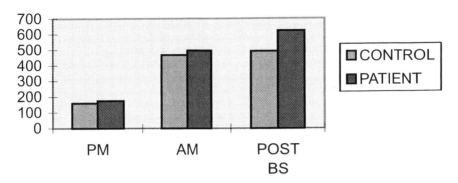

Note: Mean levels for evening, morning, and one hour after buspirone are shown for patients and controls. Bars indicate standard error.

FIGURE 3.14. Prolactin (mµ/L) Responses in CFS/ME Patients

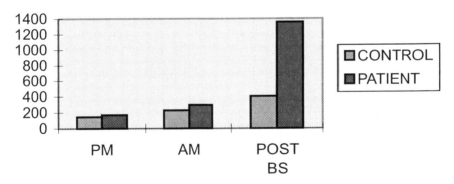

Note: Mean levels for evening, morning, and one hour after buspirone are shown for patients and controls. Bars indicate standard error.

The degree of disturbance of the sleep pattern (owl syndrome) in the patients did correlate significantly with the stimulation ratio. The owl rating was significantly different in patient and control groups. The mean value for all controls was 0.13, and for the patients it was 2.0. Three of the control subjects deliberately altered their sleep patterns for the benefit of patients, resulting in stimulation ratios much higher than those found in the remainder of the controls (see Figure 3.15).

Discussion

The number of women compared in this series does not reflect the ratio among sufferers but is weighted by those who were available to take part in this study.

Diurnal variation of cortisol secretion, which is lost in some pituitary disorders such as adenomas and compression of the brain stalk (Stewart et al., 1993), was retained in these cases. Diurnal variation of prolactin secretion was not discernible in either patients or controls. Nausea in patients as a response to buspirone was very marked in comparison to controls, and in most cases predicted the outcome of the test. Of interest also was the fact that two patients had been given paroxetine earlier for presumed depression. This is a 5-HT reuptake

FIGURE 3.15. Correlation Between Owl Syndrome Grades and Prolactin Stimulation Ratios Produced by Buspirone

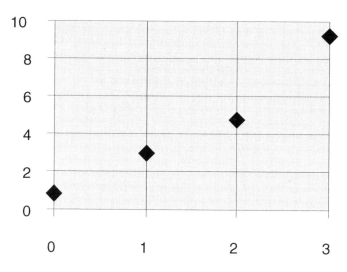

Note: Mean values ± standard error are indicated.

inhibitor with an action similar to buspirone, and in them it had produced similar nauseating effects.

The most important feature in the results is the stimulation ratio. In the patients, the mean figure for the prolactin ratio is three times higher than that in the controls, a highly significant difference. Twenty-six out of thirty patients had ratios higher than 2.5, and a similar proportion of controls had smaller ratios, assuring a reliability for the distinction of 87 percent. The cortisol stimulation ratios are higher in patients than controls, but much less so than the prolactin ratio, not achieving statistical significance for the difference between patients and controls. As such, it is an important demonstration of a biochemical abnormality in at least this group of CFS/ME patients with evidence of persistent enteroviral infection.

Although the results indicate that the hypothalamus is the chief affected site in the brain, depending on the more specific site of the lesion, symptoms vary and can affect mental function, visceral regulation, and pituitary function via the tubero-hypophyseal neurons. Although a decrease in glandular hormone secretion is possible, an increased secretion was found. However, as dopamine is the chief inhibitor of prolactin secretion, the question of a decrease in dopamine activity may be worthy of consideration; dopaminergic and serotonin (5-HT) mechanisms appear to be mutually involved. Dopamine fibers for pituitary regulation originate in the arcuate nucleus of the hypothalamus. Synthesizing neurons for dopamine itself arise in the midbrain and project to the forebrain and basal ganglia. In basal ganglia, deficits in extrapyramidal control result in Parkinsonism, while those projecting to the cortex and limbic system (meso-limbic-cortical) may be involved in psychic disturbances. Almost all neurons that synthesize 5-HT originate in the raphe nuclei of the midbrain and innervate almost all parts of the diencephalon and midbrain. Thus the nuclei for dopamine and 5-HT are in close proximity to each other. Moreover, hormonal systems have both negative and positive feedback mechanisms controlled by neuronal and biochemical means. This is seen in the hypothalamic-pituitary-adrenal axes, and many of these systems have a circadian rhythm (Meltzer, Flemming, and Robertson, 1983). Prolactin and adrenocorticotropic hormone (ACTH) secretions can be provoked by external stimuli (e.g., suckling), as well as by internal rhythmic stimuli. Dopamine is the chief prolactin inhibitor, whereas 5-HT pathways are excitatory.

The overall results as presented in this study confirm the work done by Bakheit and colleagues (1992). The studies here show that in CFS/ME patients with persistent enteroviral infection there are significant changes in hypothalamic functions. In view of more recent studies that show changes in hypothalamic blood flow in these patients, the time would seem ripe to determine what are the somatic signals that can lead a persistent virus infection to cause such changes in the brain. This in turn could open other avenues for further research into brain-body interdependence. It is also important to extend these observations to other subgroups of CFS/ME patients.

Clinical Signs

In the CNS, the long tracts are not usually remarkable except for posterior cord involvement, when temperature and touch sensations are sometimes aberrant. In the face, it is not unusual to find evidence of a segmental fifth nerve lesion, and audiometry often confirms the tensor tympani syndrome (i.e., intolerance of high frequencies). Occasionally, optical palsies, usually of the abductor muscles, are observed. Pallor of the face is fairly frequent as a feature noted by relatives and usually precedes an exacerbation of symptoms.

Other clinical signs may be found but often relate to concomitant pathology. Liver function tests are sometimes mildly abnormal and creatine phosphokinase (CPK) may be raised at rest and higher after exercise.

Tests for antibodies and viral sequences, as well as VP1, are alluded to elsewhere. If the ESR is raised, it may suggest other autoimmune or inflammatory conditions. Any concomitant illness of the same etiology, e.g., cardiac, glandular (thyroid, pancreatic, renal), etc., might be assumed to be the chief reason for the malaise.

The corollary to this is that if no concomitant illness is definable by the doctor, then it must be all in the mind! Varying hypotheses have been put forward to explain this—none of which are very convincing and can cause great distress to the patient. This has resulted in suicides in some cases, which is then seen as a verification of the original "all in the mind" diagnosis. There is conclusive evidence for the viral etiology of myocarditis in work done by L. Archard (1991) and also in pancreatitis and diabetes by Professor J. E. Banatvala and colleagues (1987), who has also investigated genetic HLA typing in these cases.

Case Report: M23

Only one case will be reported here, of a middle-aged married man with a responsible job and a happy home life. His illness commenced with a typical viral hand-foot-and-mouth disease. He had swelling of the face, eyes, and mouth and could scarcely eat or drink through a straw. He was tested for streptococcal infections, which were not found. He also had patch tests for an allergy, but none was positive. He then began to have sudden "fast feelings of movements throughout his limbs," and areas of swelling developed. His muscles began to twitch even when he was asleep, and he had considerable loss of strength and stamina—even short walks and simple tasks were exhausting, and he found it difficult to walk in a straight line. He had great difficulty in focusing, and lost two stones (13 kg) in weight from his hips, shoulders, and thighs. It appeared to be muscle loss. His breathing became difficult, and his legs, feet, and arms became quite cold, a feeling he had not previously experienced. He no longer slept through the night (owl syndrome grade 3). His doctor prescribed varying antidepressants, which were not at all helpful, although I must say that the doctors who saw him were very sympathetic.

The positive findings when I saw him included a score of 18/25 on the ME Scoring Chart, and a pericardial friction rub was present. His calf and thigh muscles had many softened areas, and, on flexing and extending the legs while seated, he displayed the usual coarse jitter seen in these cases. In the CNS, the fundi showed some hyperiemia, and he had mild bilateral nystagmus of the abducting eye. Facial sensation was poor in T1 and T2 areas on the left side, where he also had a severe tensor tympani syndrome to frequencies above 50 decibels. His long-tract reflexes were relatively normal, but he had an impaired ability to sense temperature in that heat was slow to be felt and cold produced a stinging feeling.

Serology showed high titers of coxsackie B group 1 of more than 1/512 and group 4 of 1/128. He had a positive ELISA IgM and a positive VP1 test.

Unhappily, I was told that he had terminated his life. The pathologist that performed the postmortem examination was helpful, and brain tissue that was sent to me was sent to Professor James Mowbray, who had done the previous VP1 testing. The report was as follows:

> Paraffin section from cerebral cortex; immunoperoxidase staining with monoclonal D8-1 against enteroviral VP1 protein. There is staining of protoplasm of fibroblasts around small vessels. In addition there is patchy distribution of stain in isolated glial cells throughout the section. Only a small fraction of all the glial cells is stained. Specificity confirmed by absence of staining of glial cells or perivascular fibroblasts with either normal mouse serum or a control mouse monoclonal antibody to dengue virus.
>
> DNA probe report; Enterovirus-specific cDNA probes labeled with biotin and hybridised in situ on formalin fixed and paraffin embedded 5 micron sections of autopsy material from cerebral hemispheres.
>
> Results; positive hybridisation signals were observed in the form of dense brown staining of glial cells and fibroblasts in the adventitia of normal blood vessels. No hybridisation was observed in control adjacent sections hybridised with a controlled biotin labeled vector plasmid cone.
>
> Conclusion; enterovirus specific genomic sequences were detected in this specimen indicating active infection of these cells.

We should now stop and give greater consideration to the various implications of viral infections, for they are increasing in number, severity, and diverse pathology, and it is the diverse pathology which may pose the challenge, as many are unaware of this changing pattern of disease.

Group 5

Group 5 includes those who died in my analysis and, as shown, the reasons vary (Table 3.4).

Males   26 cases out of 221 = 11.8 percent
Females   28 cases out of 457 = 6.1 percent

These statistics are self-explanatory and show an increase in malignancy in the CNS group and also confirm other reports that gliomas are much more common in the male population. Sixteen gliomas or astrocytomas have occurred over four decades in this study, following a protracted enteroviral illness that involved the central nervous system. The other carcinomas mentioned in Table 3.4 were chiefly retroperitoneal and appeared histologically to have had a pancreatic origin, and all had suffered from a previous viral pancreatitis. The cardiovascular events that were the ultimate cause of death in the CNS group were equal in both sexes.

TABLE 3.4. Cause of Death in the CNS Group

	CVS	Gliomas	Other Carcinoma	Other CNS	Suicide	SSPE
Males	6	12	2	3	1	2
%	2.7	5.4	0.9	1.35	0.45	0.9
Females	11	4	0	8	2	3
%	2.4	0.9	0	1.75	0.44	0.66

Chapter 4

Familial Consequences
of Viral Illness

The term familial, as used here, is not meant to specify an illness that is necessarily genetic in character, but rather an illness or a sequence of illnesses which may occur over years and appear to have a common origin. Such an illness may affect one individual and have ongoing consequences while the other family members escape, or it may run a course at varying intervals of time in one member, or other members may subsequently develop a syndrome with a similar etiology. This series is confined to the long-term study of families in which virus infection has been a problem. No doubt the study could be applied to other areas, such as occupational hazards (e.g., lead, asbestos or exposure to insecticides, etc.). However, this study, which included a diversity of occupations and a range of patient ages, from intrapartum to maturity, was confined to viral etiological factors. This should not be taken to mean that other factors could not have an effect, and indeed an inquiring mind would wish to know why some isolated individuals succumb and the rest of the family remain well, while in other cases other members of the same family succumb.

This chapter briefly summarizes some of the material from a prospective study that began in embryonic form forty years ago. It has gathered both momentum and significance over the years and involves an in-depth study of more than 450 families. The families entered the study for one of two reasons. In the first case, one member had an ongoing sequential illness following proven viral infection. The illness did not remit within six months but caused ongoing pathology in one organ, e.g., heart, kidney, or pancreas; such patients made up Group 3 in the series. Where more than one organ was affected they entered Group 4, which includes multiorgan pathology.

The second reason to join the study was that in some families another member became ill, or a previously affected member, who had apparently recovered within the specified six-month period, succumbed a second time and did not recover within the six-month period. These members would then enter Groups 3 or 4. Thus a family pattern began to emerge that could be seen by a family doctor who looked for it, and its relationship to the individual and family could be more completely investigated.

ANECDOTAL CASE STUDIES

Here I present only ten cases, selected more or less at random, to illustrate the family groups studied. A few cases are presented in more depth in other chapters on specific syndromes, but in this section the patients are seen in relation to other members of the same family. It is appropriate to mention that, because of marriage, family names may change. For this reason, in hospital practice certain cases in this series were seen with similar illnesses, and the family relationship was never noted. In some cases a family member was admitted with an illness and weeks later another member of the family but of the opposite sex was admitted with an identical illness, but into a different ward, and no connection was observed.

In one family, a mother was admitted because of a violent headache, and a lumbar puncture was performed to exclude a possible subarachnoid hemorrhage. No hemorrhage was found, and the diagnosis was viral meningoencephalitis. A week or so later her son was admitted with an identical illness. He also had a lumbar puncture because of the same tentative diagnosis. The outcome was the same. The family relationship was not observed by the hospital medical staff. Thus, as in other cases, both the immediate and the longitudinal studies are more within the orbit of the family doctor. The actual reason for consequential illnesses may lie in family genetics or family infection, or both. We may then question what this means, or attempt to draw some tentative conclusions from the study. It may be appro-

priate to begin with those in whom congenital abnormalities have occurred as an apparent sequel to infection.

Family 01

A family of three. Their baby (referred to as case F22) was born in
1975. At the time of conception, the mother had a Bornholm disease
type of illness. The father is included in Chapter 2 (M11) and died with a
cardiomyopathy shortly after the baby was born. His titers were 1/256
for coxsackie B group 2 and 1/128 for coxsackie B group 4, but a stool
culture was positive, and he had a positive, IgM and IgG serology also.
His chest X ray is shown in Chapter 2 and photographs of the child are in
Chapter 3. The photo of the child as a baby shows a large mouth and
flabby, rather fat limbs, which may be considered healthy, but as shown,
the large mouth persisted in later years. Chromosome analysis and many
tests were unrevealing. Amyotonia congenita appears to be the term that
covers the syndrome, as she had muscle degeneration, and at fifteen
years of age was tube fed and unable to sit up in bed. She died shortly after the last photograph (Figure 3.2) was taken. The question is whether
the mother had a first-trimester infection, indicated by the baby's large
mouth, or maybe a later infection while the baby was in utero. A later
pregnancy was normal, suggesting infection in utero in this case. Thus,
both father and daughter died, the father from a comparatively short, serious illness and the daughter from a prolonged, fifteen-year deteriorat-
ing illness. Without careful studies at the time these two would not be
seen as having a common etiology cause.

Family 02

A family of two until a male baby was born in 1987. At the time of
conception this baby's mother, twenty-three years old, had a coxsackie infection, reported February 1987, and her last period was the
same week. She had typical Bornholm disease, and her titers showed
a fourfold rise in coxsackie B groups 3 and 5 and a positive ELISA
IgM. The illness did not appear to be severe and could easily have
been considered "just a virus" and not connected with the subsequent
outcome in the baby. However, in view of the infection I monitored
the baby carefully, and in the early weeks of life he appeared to be un-

responsive to light. A videotape shows his unresponsiveness to light and movement, but a good response to tactile and auditory sensations. Later, the MRI scan (Figure 4.1) was performed, which shows the agenesis of the septum pellucidum. He is now a fine little boy, very happy, musically oriented, and rapidly acquiring the ability to read Braille. He brings much happiness to the family. A subsequent pregnancy was normal, as in the other cases, suggesting in utero infection in the first trimester.

Family 03

A family of two until the advent of the baby. This female was born at thirty-eight weeks gestation, and the mother had a clinical viral Bornholm disease in the first trimester with a significant rise in titers. The birth was uneventful, but subsequent progress was slow. I explained to the mother that I felt that myelination had not fully taken place, but suggested that maybe in the immediate future it might oc-

FIGURE 4.1. MRI Showing Agenesis of the Septum Pellucidum

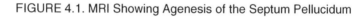
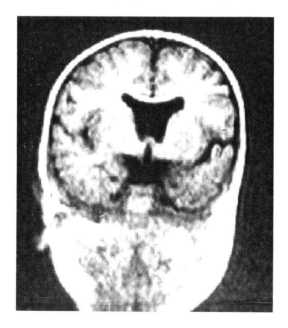

cur. However, this hope did not materialize. Again, MRI scanning was done, and the report on the brain imaging is as follows: "There was a symmetrical pattern of myelination, but there were abnormal signals surrounding the trigones, sparing the frontal horns. The bodies of the lateral ventricles were enlarged." The scans show a general paucity of white matter and confirm the clinical impression of a lack of myelination development (see Figure 4.2). This child was also videotaped for future reference and is quite severely retarded. Later, another conception occurred, and a boy was born who appeared normal. However, in his early years he also had a coxsackie meningitis and had epilepsy with an abnormal EEG response, but recovered well. The epilepsy has not continued. In my series, 80 percent of children who have epilepsy with a febrile illness do in fact recover, but in childhood are more prone to convulsions if another illness occurs. This susceptibility to epileptic-type seizures appears to remit with maturity in most cases.

FIGURE 4.2. MRI Scans Showing Paucity of White Matter, Confirming Lack of Myelination Development

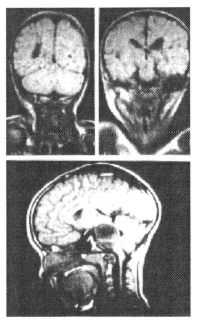

Family 04

A family of four. The mother, thirty-five years old, had viral meningitis in 1979 with rising titers of coxsackie B group 4 in the 1/1000 range. The family consisted of the parents and two children, a male and a female. The family was tested and found to have raised levels of coxsackie B group 4 in all members, but only the mother was ill. The illness terminated without sequel but in 1982 recurred, and again the titers rose to more than 1/1000. On this occasion the mother was pregnant, and a male baby was delivered and appeared normal. After carefully monitoring the baby, a cardiac murmur was found at about ten weeks of age. A pediatric colleague saw the baby and postulated that he had a congenital valve lesion. As I had watched the baby carefully from birth, this was not convincing, and his subsequent progress was downhill. He went into failure despite care and died before he was a year old. The photograph shows the massive endocardial fibroelastosis that had developed (see Figure 4.3).

FIGURE 4.3. Endocardial Fibroelastosis

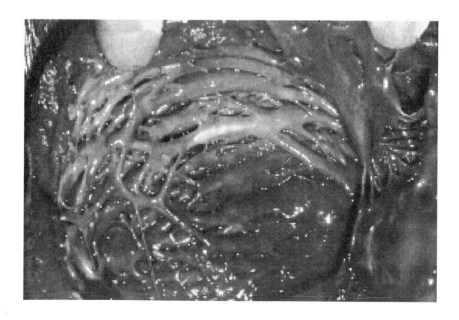

Once again, the whole family's titers were checked, and again coxsackie group 4 showed a general rise, but no other member was ill. However, five years later, the other son, who by then was seventeen years old, presented at the surgery with a short history of a feeling of chest oppression and some dyspnea (discussed previously as case M04). After examination and electrocardiography, a diagnosis of viral myocarditis was made. His serological titers once more showed a fourfold rise, and he had a positive ELISA IgM. He also had a rise to 1/128 in the adenoviral group, the significance of which is not certain, for no other member of the family was affected and he had no apparent lymphadenopathy. His subsequent progress was stormy, and he had to have a heart transplant. After this his titers of cytomegalovirus rose to 1/512, no doubt due to the immune suppression therapy. His VP1 antigen test became markedly positive also. This family is a very good example of the ongoing effects of viral illness within a family, affecting different members. The casual observer or specialist would not be in a position to relate these events and illnesses to a common source.

Family 05

Family 05 consisted of a mother, father, and a child, all of whom were healthy. The mother became pregnant in the early part of 1970. In the last trimester she had chest pain, and her ECG showed myocarditis. She was seen by myself and one of my late cardiological consultants who took an interest in this type of case. Myocarditis was confirmed in subsequent in-depth investigations, and also ECHO strain virus was cultured from her stools. The baby was delivered but was stillborn, and autopsy showed a flabby heart, which was diagnostic of myocarditis. Following this in the same year, the husband was ill with severe pain of the Bornholm type, and he had an eightfold rise in coxsackie B group 4. He later also developed pancreatitis and within two years developed insulin-dependent diabetes. After approximately another two years, he began to lose weight, and a retroperitoneal mass was found at laparoscopy, which histologically was shown to be a carcinoma of the pancreas. The family moved out of the area, but I was able to follow his progress, which was protracted. He eventually died from this carcinoma.

Family 06

Family 06 consisted of a father, mother, and two sons. The father developed Bornholm disease and his titers of Coxsackievirus rose to 1/512 for group 5 and 1/128 for group 4. He also had a positive ELISA IgM. He developed pancreatitis identical to the father in the previous case, except that he did not develop diabetes. His wife also had raised titers of the same strain of virus and later developed thyroid antibodies, which, as discussed in Chapter 5, is more prevalent in females; she also developed pernicious anemia. Later she required thyroxin therapy for mild thyroid failure. Some four years later the father developed a carcinoma of the pancreas, from which he died. His son married, moved away, and had a daughter who is now a woman. Two years after his father died, he also had Bornholm disease, and his titers were identical to his father's in groups 4 and 5 of coxsackie B. He also had a positive ELISA IgM and a positive IgG and VP1. Like his father, he developed pancreatitis and was admitted several times to the hospital with exacerbations. So far he is well, and only time will reveal if there will be more serious consequences. His father was a teetotaler, and the son only rarely drank alcohol. The daughter has also had quite severe Bornholm disease, and her titers were 1/1000 to groups 4 and 5 coxsackie B. She also had a positive ELISA IgM. She has not had any further sequelae, however. This family has been followed up since the 1970s. As with other families, serial titers have been assessed over many years, and it is interesting that it has taken seven years for the daughter's titers to fall, and her father's still show a positive VP1 at this writing.

Family 07

This elderly couple had been ballroom dancers and very healthy, but in 1977, in their sixties, they demonstrated a startling sequence of family illness that could not be ignored. The husband suddenly became ill and was seen by myself and Dr. H. A. Dewar. He had a viral myocarditis. His titers of coxsackie B group 4 rose to over 1/512, and he had a positive culture and also positive ELISA IgM and later IgG. His ECG was typical, with ST segment elevations and N-shaped configurations in varying chest leads from day to day. He had a very stormy time and spent several months in bed, as the deleterious effects of exercise in this condition have been well demonstrated in mice as well as humans. He gradually improved, but many weeks later he had a severe peritoneal reaction and also developed massive orchitis. It was so hard that a biopsy was done to rule out malignancy. The orchitis eventually resolved completely. He then developed pancreatitis, which resolved after a fairly difficult illness. Later still he began to have pain with abnormal signs in the right iliac fossa (RIF). An appendectomy was performed and an isolated carcinoma in situ of the appendix was removed, and all gland biopsies were negative. He made an uneventful recovery.

During his recovery in 1979, his wife was found collapsed in the garden, and it was thought that she was dead. However, she was not, but an ECG showed a myocarditis similar to her husband's. Her titers were identical to his, as were the ELISA IgM and IgG, but we did not culture any virus. She had a challenging passage, being confined to bed for months. She also developed pancreatitis and had bilateral pelvic pain suggestive of oophoritis. She gradually recovered, and for a year or more they had a moderately peaceful life.

The husband then began to lose weight and complained of back pain. On investigation, once again a carcinoma of the pancreas was demonstrated, from which he later died. Two or three years later his wife began to lose height and showed signs of osteoporosis. She was admitted to a nursing home. However, two years after the move she began to have signs and symptoms resembling those of her husband, and she also died of carcinoma of the pancreas. Neither ever showed signs of diabetes. This may be relevant, as in this series a diabetic outcome is more often found in young people.

Family 08

Family 08 consisted of a man, wife, and daughter. The father was born in 1926 and was seen in 1965 having severe Bornholm disease with pain in the abdomen and in the back, suggestive of pancreatitis. A week later he had chest pain, and a PFR and ECG showed perimyocarditis. He had titers of 1/512 for coxsackie B group 4 and also a positive ELISA IgM and later IgG. His complement fell to 50 percent. He gradually recovered but developed a non-insulin-dependent diabetes. He also developed a radiculopathy of the shoulder girdle with wasting of the periscapular muscles. During the following years, his daughter, who was born in 1953, had a Bornholm disease. She married and had a baby but later, in 1984, had a recurrence and also pericarditis. Her titers, similar to her father's, rose to more than 1/512 for coxsackie B group 4 and groups 1, 2, 3, and 5 also showed a rise to 1/64. She had a positive ELISA IgM and later a positive IgG. About this time she became pregnant and was booked under my care for hospital delivery. Unfortunately, I was not called until after the baby was born and, on arrival, I found that it had died. I examined the baby's body and discovered a very large liver. Subsequent examination suggested viral myocarditis, which was confirmed at autopsy. A few years later, when the myocarditis had subsided and her titers fell, the daughter had another pregnancy, which progressed normally, and the baby was normal. Her father, however, died a year or two after this due to a retroperitoneal carcinoma which appeared to have a pancreatic origin.

Family 09

Family 09 comprised a couple in their thirties whose illness began in 1972. The husband had titers of coxsackie B groups 3 and 4 of 1/1000 and groups 5 and 6 of 1/32, a positive ELISA IgM and IgG, as well as a positive stool culture. He later developed leukemia and died. Years later his widow became ill and had perimyocarditis with similar titers and also a positive ELISA IgM and IgG and a positive culture. Later still, a chest X ray showed a linear mass in the mediastinum that at operation proved to be a dermoid cyst about 10 cm long. It is my view that this was possibly due to an embryonic remnant that had been stimulated to cell division by the virus. Her subsequent progress was downhill, and she developed severe myalgic encephalomyelitis. This diagnosis was not accepted by her family at the time, and she transferred to another doctor and later spent a long time in a psychiatric hospital, where she lost weight and made no progress. She returned to my care after two or more years, and a videotape was made of her rather sad state at the time—it is invaluable now. Further tests were done, and her VP1 test proved to be highly positive. Treatment was begun with high doses of gamma globulin, though I had some reservations because of the lapse of time. Within months, however, she was out of her bed and dressed. At this writing she has put on four stones (25 kg) in weight and is enjoying some social life. However, she developed some skin lesions, which also have been photographed (Figure 4.4). Histologically they are mycosis fungoides. They appear to have remitted, as she has improved with treatment, but it is too early to envisage the eventual outcome.

Family 10

Family 10 consisted of a father, mother, daughter, and son. This family history began in 1953. The father was then in his early forties and had an acute viral chest illness and also myocarditis and encephalitis. His titers of coxsackie B group 4 rose to 1/512, and he had a positive culture. His complement fell dramatically, and he developed a positive IgM and IgG response later. He was initially very ill and confused his doctors by complaining of inverted vision, which some

FIGURE 4.4. Granuloma Fungoides

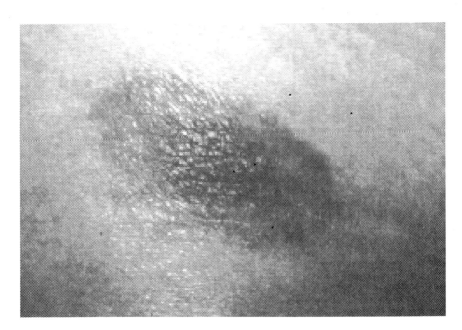

considered hysterical. Through the years his vision improved, but he was never able to focus well afterward. These vision disturbances are seen in the ME group often and will be discussed elsewhere. The cardiac condition appeared to resolve, but he developed cardiomegally and also angina and eventually had to have coronary artery surgery. The coronary arteries were stenosed, but without atheroma as in other cases described in Chapter 2. This is similar to the pathology seen in mitral stenosis. He deteriorated considerably later and died due to a severe cardiomyopathy and heart failure.

The son was born in 1952 and in 1970 became ill in a similar way. He also had a rise in coxsackie B virus group 4, to 1/512, and again, like his father, had a positive IgM and later IgG and a positive culture. He had a marked myocarditis, and one cardiologist wondered whether it was due to alcohol, as he drove the brewery van—but he did not drink! However, in view of the unfounded suspicion, he was subjected to a needle biopsy of the liver, which showed a well-marked vasculitis, which I have demonstrated in a few other cases of coxsackie B virus infection. The biopsy has been repeated for diverse reasons in both males and females, and a similar vasculitis noted. However, in his case it did not show the signs of alcoholism. Over the years he has recovered and so far remains fairly well.

CONCLUSION

It is obvious that these anecdotal cases can only generally suggest the varying syndromes seen in other families. The conclusion to be drawn might be that this is how families normally die, which would be erroneous. Most of the families showed a marked rise of antibody titers in unaffected members who never became ill, which is dealt with again in Chapter 6. However, there are sufficient families whose members are severely affected to make more research rewarding, and the family doctor is in a unique position to do it, given the ambition and time.

It should be remarked once again that marriage can cause confusion due to name changes. Three sisters in this series had different marital names. One was referred to me due to the late effects of viral illness while the other two were under my care. One of the latter had severe myalgic encephalomyelitis and the other had a marked viral myocarditis as did the sister who had been referred. Both of the patients with myocarditis died due to dysrhythmias, and the ME victim sadly took her own life. She washed, dressed, powdered herself, lay on an immaculately tidy bed, placed a sprig of roses on her chest, and, after taking tablets, folded her arms across her chest and expired. In a similar case referred to in Chapter 3 as case M23, the brain was examined carefully and virus was demonstrated.

Many variables can confuse the observers, such as change of name and location. Allowing for these restrictions, the illnesses that occur in families do point toward environmental and host factors which warrant consideration.

The family represented in Figure 4.5 illustrates the common etiology of infection that almost certainly is the cause of the illnesses to which varying members succumbed over three generations. The titers for enteroviruses, in these cases all CBV group 4, are still retained, and the VP1 later became positive. The child who had mesangial nephropathy died while waiting for a suitable kidney donor. At autopsy, he also was shown to have an agenesis of the left kidney. He was in his early thirties when he died.

FIGURE 4.5. Family Tree Illustrating the Common Etiology of Infection

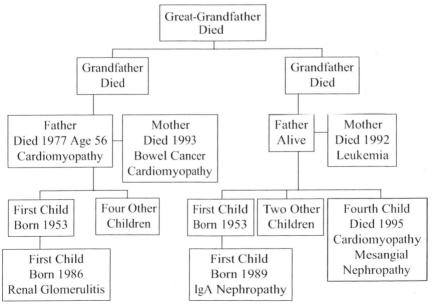

Chapter 5

Glandular and Other
Organ Syndromes

Glandular syndromes in this series of 1,800 cases occurred in 107 females (5.9 percent of all cases) and in 104 males (5.7 percent of all cases). Other concomitant pathology frequently exists, e.g., a CVS or CNS syndrome.

The lungs, kidneys, stomach, and bowel are all considered in this chapter, as biologically they have a specialized physiological role. The lymph glands are included along with the familiar exocrine and endocrine glands such as the thyroid, pancreas, thymus, and also the pineal gland. It is worthy of notice that the hypothalamus, as referred to in Chapter 3, also plays a vital mediating role in some syndromes that otherwise would be considered the result of a more specific, localized gland dysfunction.

Before describing case histories, an overview of the basis of hormone regulatory function might be helpful. For example, polypetide hormones, are a diverse set of regulatory molecules that convey information, not only from cell to cell, but also from organ to organ throughout the body. They act as neurotransmitters in the central, autonomic, and peripheral systems for the purpose of organ-to-organ communication. It should be remembered that the same neurohormone acting on varying organ receptors will produce an effect that is not in keeping with the hormone itself, but is in keeping with the function of the organ that is either stimulating or inhibiting. Most of these hormones are the result of the cleavage of precursors found within the Golgi complex. The hormones are then transported to the membrane of the cell. A change in extracellular homeostasis results and causes the appropriate hormone release, which, when it binds to a receptor site, either changes the receptor or acts on the receptor by changing it from an inactive to an active form as a molecule. This then has an affinity for other binding sites—and so the chain reaction proceeds.

Mineralocorticoids are a good example, for they regulate the electrolyte balance in the kidney, salivary, and sweat glands as well as those of the GI tract. Receptors for steroid hormones are found in the brain, in particular in the hypothalamus and pituitary gland. Thus steroids act on and regulate the hypothalamic-hypophysial system producing various effects, among which is the regulation of the reproductive system. For example, glucocorticoids in this area control the release of ACTH by the excretion of cortisol-releasing factor.

Other metabolic processes that are regulated include, and are as diverse as, cell reproduction and differentiation. Thus, physiological communication and harmony depend on endocrine, paracrine, and autocrine function, as well as on the function of the neurotransmitters, which are not only central but also peripheral to the furthest part of the body. Circulatory changes from the most central to the most peripheral areas are a simple example. In humans at least a hundred hormones are known to be involved at these levels. Again, some are inhibitory and some are stimulatory on cell receptors, and the ultimate balance is determined not only by this, but also by the ongoing chain reaction that results, when other cell receptors are affected, as shown earlier. Also, some receptors are in the cytoplasm (e.g., for steroids), while others are on the cell membrane (e.g., for the neurotransmitters). This is interesting because antibodies can act on and neutralize the effects of hormones on these receptor sites.

An example of this action is the antibody that can act on the insulin receptor site of a cell and thereby render the patient insulin resistant. Also, in some cases of postviral-mediated syndromes, antithyroid antibodies have occasionally been shown to have a similar effect. These hormones act on the cell membrane and thus are accessible to any antibody at the time of its biological action. It is interesting that hormones such as steroids, which, as mentioned, are within the cytoplasm, are not so easily affected. One other example of membrane-blocking activity might conceivably occur in myasthenia gravis, four cases of which have followed viral infection in this series. This illustrates one of the pathological effects of the virus on the thymus, but other diverse glandular effects occur which almost certainly include those affecting the pineal body.

The pineal gland, so called because it resembles a pinecone, is a neurohormonal secretory gland. To a certain extent it is regulated by light via the suprachiasmatic nucleus, which receives nerve impulses from the retina. Crucial to the regulation of pineal function is a sympathetic nerve supply of noradrenergic fibers. The pineal gland is not subject to the blood-brain barrier. The pinealocytes are regulated by beta-adrenergic receptors, and thus blocking of these or section of the sympathetic innovation inhibits pineal function. Pineal functions can affect the timing of puberty, and melatonin has a significant role in this effect. Other amines found in the pineal gland include norepinephrin, serotonin, histamine, and dopamine together with LH-RH, TRH, somatostatin, and an analog of oxytocin. GABA is also found in the pineal gland. This is an inhibitory neurotransmitter. Melatonin is synthesized from tryptophan. At night, during darkness, melatonin secretion is highest, and its precursor, serotonin, is low. Melatonin inhibits gonadotropin secretion when it reaches the hypothalamus and pituitary gland. It also induces sleepiness, particularly REM sleep, but, oddly, in depressed patients this function is impaired. Further effects of melatonin are discussed in Chapter 1.

However, it should be remembered that the hormones which act internally within the cell have an effect on the membrane. To complicate matters, there are also antireceptor antibodies distinct from the hormone antibody, and these antibodies can recognize the areas of receptors that are separate from the hormone-binding domain. The numbers of receptors also varies with the specificity of the cell—maybe from 100 to 1 million. Furthermore, it has been shown in the case of beta-blockers that as one site is blocked the cell may produce more receptors, and only the surface area available limits this continuing process. Thus the target cell number of binding sites is consistent with the requirements of the endocrine system, or perhaps is modified by other means. Thus it can be seen that the binding of molecules on the cell surface in minute amounts relays messages to sites within the cell, or vice versa. Molecules on the cell surface might affect the "household function" of the cell with its immediate relay to other organs and cells, while within the cell the whole metabolism and function of the cell would be affected. This latter consequence could be defined as an autocrine effect.

Apart from this blocking mechanism, physiological changes within the cell membrane may occur, e.g., its phospholipid content can inhibit or augment the receptor function with its transmembrane signal effect, and conceivably this is why the use of essential fatty acids can be helpful. They are essential membrane constituents, and a brief résumé of their function is as follows:

1. They act on receptors and membrane enzymes.
2. They act as messengers after the following chain-reaction conversion:
    a. *Linoleic acid.* A genetic dysfunction may occur here that may prevent the normal desaturation to:
    b. *Gammalinoleic acid.* This in turn desaturates to:
    c. *Dihomogammalinoleic acid.* This is converted to eicosanoids. Interferon activity commences here.
    d. *Prostaglandins* are the result of formation by the cyclooxygenase system.

Interferon activity may be inhibited if linoleic acid is not converted to the gammalinoleic form or if cyclooxygenase is lacking and therefore the interferon activity through prostoglandins is inhibited.

As mentioned earlier, the number of receptors on a cell surface may vary for several reasons, and generally there are "spare receptors" on the cell membrane. A loss of these, or a downregulation of their functional ability, may also be due to a diminished sensitivity to bind the requisite hormone or to a diminished sensitivity to the bound hormone. The former may be overcome by additional hormone administration, as in one case where there was evidence of lack of ability to bind T4, and its augmented administration resulted in distinct improvement. The block in functional ability was more seriously demonstrated in one patient in the hospital, who went into an insulin-resistant phase and died despite the use of 4,000 units of insulin. This case will be referred to again later.

These considerations have a widespread significance for pathology, for no single hormone has a simple or single effect. After integrating with a receptor, the result may be an interaction with other effector systems, and so a synergistic or antagonistic effect will be produced. In addition, an excess of hormone can lead to ultimate degradation of receptors and eventually to an actual decrease in receptor numbers. This may be the reason for so-called insulin resistance. Also, I have noted clinically that, when using steroids for severe intercranial arteritis or IgG for viral myocarditis, if the treatment is discontinued before total cure of the pathology, the reintroduction of the treatment can meet with a very refractory host response. It seems logical to relate this to receptor-hormone uptake, and obviously this could be helpful in some circumstances as well as adverse in others. This does not make the problem simple.

In the neurohypophysis, the tracts are unmyelinated, and the principal secretions are arginine vasopressin (AVP) and oxytocin as well as TRH and CRH. It is of interest that, in the cases of virus-mediated CNS illness affecting the hypothalamus, some of the paraventricular cells are in association with the brain stem and cord and others with the areas that are associated with emotion and other functions such as memory. In the cord they have an effect on the autonomic system. In the brain stem they are in contact with the vagus and the ninth cranial nerve and thereby play a role in the control of blood pressure and bowel activity.

It is thus interesting to view the body as one whole that interrelates and works together, and not as separate "pieces." The atria of the heart provide an example, for they are often considered mere lobbies to the ventricles, although the left atrium has endocrine control of blood volume mediated through atrial natriuretic peptides (ANP) in its muscle cells. The muscle cells react to tension by secretion of the Aps, which act on the renal tubules and stimulate the excretion of sodium, which in turn modulates blood volume. This is an interesting synergistic link between organs as separate as the kidney and left atrium. There are also receptors in the third ventricle of the brain that are sensitive to these atrial peptides. Here the ANPs inhibit AVP release, which in turn inhibits the desire to drink. In summary, this is a picture of the way in which the peripheral and central neural systems are integrated for the defense of the whole body.

There is also an interaction between emotional stress, which might be due to illness, and external factors—but in both, AVP is released due to the stress situation. Thus vasopressin and plasma osmolality, together with thirst, are all regulated by the hypothalamus; conversely, feedback from renal angiotensin into the hypothalamus will stimulate thirst. Via the same pathway, the effects of stress can also result in the inhibition of micturition and also the production of breast milk. The perivascular spaces in this area have fenestrations that are seen in other glands and no doubt serve a purpose, for the modulation of effects similar to that seen in the renal glomerulus and its surrounding nephron.

These perivascular, infiltrated spaces sometimes are evident as so-called UBOs on MRI scans and have been noted by myself and others in some cases of myalgic encephalomyelitis. It is in this area, and affecting the pituitary, that regulation of such hormones as ACTH and prolactin occurs. Dopamine appears to be the main prolactin release-inhibitory factor. There are also other inhibitory and release factors for growth hormone (GH) and TSH. As shown earlier, one hormone may exert several effects synergistically; e.g., TRH can also release prolactin and GH and ACTH in certain circumstances. Although dopamine is the chief inhibitor of prolactin, it can also inhibit TSH and GH. TRH, on the other hand, acts by stimulating-prolactin releasing factor, which in turn releases prolactin. Perhaps I can summarize by saying that the main effect of the hypothalamus on prolactin is inhibition, but among the prolactin stimulants are hormones such as TRH, AVP, vasoactive intestinal peptide (VIP), and oxytocin.

Dopamine itself has diverse functions and is synthesized mainly by cells in the midbrain and others in the forebrain. Those that project to the basal ganglia have an extrapyramidal control and are involved in Parkinson's disease, while those projecting to the mesolimbic cortical area may be involved in schizophrenia. In this series, in the 1950s a number of cases developed acute schizophrenia after a viral illness. Most of these recovered fully after a short illness. The Leeds group (Peatfield, 1987) also described subcortical dementia as a postviral syndrome. As stated, dopamine appears to be the chief inhibitor of prolactin secretion, and the main effect of the hypothalamus on prolactin is suppression. In the tests we have done using buspirone in ME cases, there is an apparent stimulation of prolactin by the drug. Thus neurotransmitted impulses that stimulate the hypothalamus will suppress prolactin via dopaminergic pathways, while the serotonin pathways are excitatory. Therefore, the explanation for the changes in prolactin secretion due to buspirone is rather complex.

Here I would simply make the comment and await further research for the explanation of the changes (see Figure 5.1).

However, to sum up these mechanisms, it can be said that the effect of a hormone on a cell results in a response which is the result of that particular cell's function rather than that of the hormone itself. This response may be upregulated or downregulated. This also may be due to, or modified by, the effects of a self-regulatory mechanism, or by a drug such as a monoamine oxidase inhibitor. If the self-regulatory mechanism is suppressed, then the resultant response may be not only an upregulation but also a hypersensitivity to other factors such as food or drugs (e.g., cheese). Reviewing the cell-mediated response via its membrane activity, it becomes obvious that this may be blocked by an antibody or a chemical such as a beta-blocker. Of course, these are only examples of multitudinous causes and effects at this cellular level.

Thus, we can say that organ-specific diseases are due to organ-specific antibodies, autoantibodies, or direct viral attack. On the other hand, glands may be involved in an illness, but the antibodies are not organ specific. Case F34 is a good example, for a needle biopsy demonstrated vasculitis of the liver, but the serum showed mitochondrial and parietal cell antibodies that were not specific to the liver. She had also developed diabetes, which was very poorly controlled by therapy. Hypothetically, the diabetes, as with other diseases, could be shown to be not only a primary glandular cell dysfunction but also an end organ cell receptor dysfunction. It should be apparent that the end organ receptor for insulin, etc., must be configuratively specific for insulin, as also are the terminal receptors for thyroxin, acetylcholine, etc. That these can be "blocked" by some other substance is clearly shown by the chain action of beta-blockers.

In the case of the woman who entered an insulin-resistant phase and died despite receiving 4,000 units of insulin, she was found in an unconscious state one morning, and clinically it seemed that this could have been due to hypoglycemia as she was insulin dependent, and the early stages of her diabetes had been difficult to control. Intravenous dextrose, however, produced no improvement whatsoever. She was transferred immediately to a hospital, and her serological tests showed a high glucose level and all the clinical signs of hypo-

FIGURE 5.1. Response to Stress

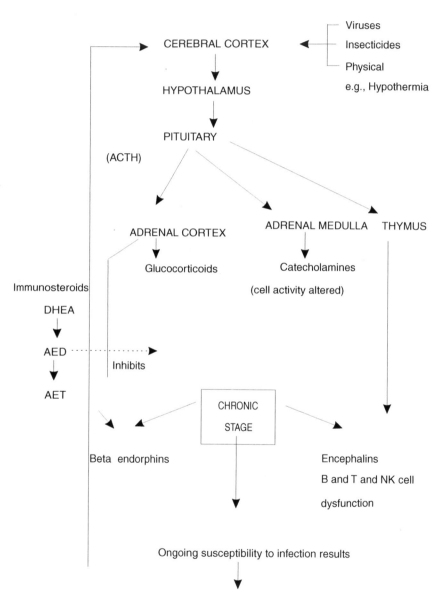

insulinemia. The consensus of opinion was that this was due to end organ receptor block. It is interesting to ask if she may have had some response to sulfonylureas, which stimulate the end organ receptors; or perhaps to steroids, which could have modified the autoimmune antibody-blocking response. In this case, autoantibodies mimicking insulin and blocking the end organ receptor could theoretically have been responsible and might have been modified by steroids. It is a concept that should be borne in mind, not only for the diabetic, but also by extrapolation for other glandular syndromes.

This process could be further illustrated by a case, F31, who developed thyroid antibodies. She was clinically stabilized on 0.3 mg thyroxin per day. Her T4 was rather high but lower doses of thyroxin rendered her clinically hypothyroid. The evidence suggested end organ receptor block. She is currently maintained and is well on 0.3 mg thyroxin. There is evidence that this can occur also in some, but not all, cases of myasthenia gravis, and the concept opens up a field of investigation in other, more remote areas of apparent gland-mediated syndromes. Thus, it would be wise to always consider the functions of both the propagating cell and the receptor as a physiological unit. The possible mechanism is shown in Figure 5.2, with an anti-idiotypic response. The sequence is as follows:

- Virus attachment to organ cell membrane
- Antibody formation
- Memory cell receptor typing
- Other lymphocyte antibody formation to the memory cell antibody image

This idiotypic formation of antibodies would be acceptable to the end organ receptor and act as a blocking agent in its own right, thus excluding the attachment of the native molecule, with or without subsequent cell destruction. The oral medications for diabetes are known to have an effect on the end organ receptors and either "free" the blocked receptors or stimulate the formation of new receptor areas. This would fit in with the concept that not all the pathology of diabetes is due solely to insulin depletion.

When considering all the cases, it becomes obvious that many syndromes are not isolated but are part of a pattern in the patient in which glandular pathology is also evident. As in other cases, there is a ten-

FIGURE 5.2. Molecular Mimicry and Autoimmune Illness

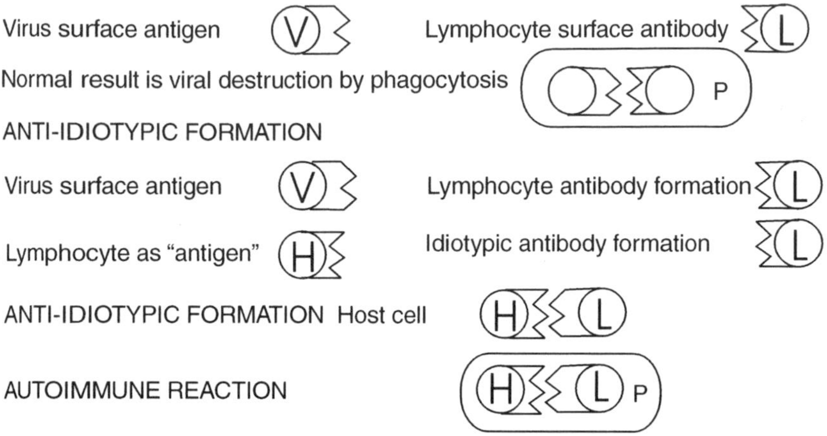

Virus surface antigen   (V)   Lymphocyte surface antibody (L)

Normal result is viral destruction by phagocytosis   (⟨⟩ ⟨⟩ P)

ANTI-IDIOTYPIC FORMATION

Virus surface antigen   (V)   Lymphocyte antibody formation (L)

Lymphocyte as "antigen"   (H)   Idiotypic antibody formation   (L)

ANTI-IDIOTYPIC FORMATION   Host cell   (H) (L)

AUTOIMMUNE REACTION   ((H) (L) P)

dency to treat these syndromes in isolation or as merely additional, whereas it can be clearly shown that it is much more accurate to consider them as part of the whole disease process. This disease process could occur due to the effects of the virus on the gland itself, as seen in the pancreas of a diabetic mouse, but even this is not simple, for it has been shown that an isolated pancreas infected by coxsackie B group 4 still produces insulin, whereas in the mouse model there is islet cell necrosis. The latter is due not to the virus itself, but to the activity of the NK cells of the host, which attack the virus-infected cells; or it may be the effects of the resultant autoimmune process, as discussed in the previous paragraphs, and may occur early or as a late manifestation after the initial infection. Thus an excess of suppressor cells has been deemed abnormal, whereas it really is part of host protection—it is better to protect virus-infected cells, even if they are "sick" and their function is impaired, than to lyse all of them resulting in ultimate organ destruction. Therefore, the "central" organ or also its copartner, the end organ receptor, can be primarily affected.

It should be stated here that sequelae are not organ specific and yet affect several organs. A number of odd antibodies have been found in this series, some of which can react with DNA and other nuclear elements. Thus, in this series, about 25 percent of patients, mainly females, who had antithyroid antibodies also had parietal cell antibodies, and antinuclear antibodies have been found in others also. The fact that a number of organs are affected could be attributed to a type of autoimmune systemic vasculitis that can ensue. Hence in the renal cases reported, some of which had a needle biopsy, the lesion was shown to be a glomerulitis that did not affect the nephron, similar to the hepatic vasculitic lesion referred to earlier. This can be conceptualized as a spectrum where at one end there appear to be organ-specific antibodies to one organ and at the other end multifactorial elements, of which systemic vasculitis is a good example.

In some cases it may appear that only one end organ is affected, yet in other cases, such as diabetes, it is apparent from the optic syndromes and the peripheral arteritis with gangrene that sometimes occur, as well as the neurological and renal sequelae, that this is a multifactorial autoimmune disease, linked perhaps by a systemic vasculitis, or an autoimmune connective tissue disorder. In mutant mice some cases show a possible genetic predisposition, but this is not the only factor. Professor Loria (1986a) has shown the effects of viral infection, which in the DB/DB homozygote will cause islet cell necrosis and diabetes without inflammation, while in the DB/db heterozygote diabetes occurs with inflammation. In the former there is a lack of organ-specific antibodies but many NK cells, while in the latter such antibodies are present and account for the inflammatory response. The host effects of a pancreas infected with coxsackie B group 4 are shown in Table 5.1.

In systemic lupus erythematosus (SLE), for example, the so-called LE cell is formed by polymorphs that ingest other white blood cells

TABLE 5.1. Host Effects of Coxsackie B Group 4-Infected Pancreas

Genetics	Necrosis	Inflammation	Antibodies
DB/DB			
Islet	++	—	—
Acinar	++	—	
DB/+			
Islet	++	—	+
Acinar	—	—	
+/+			
Islet	—	++	++
Acinar	—	++	

(WBCs), that in turn contain antibodies that bind complement by having bonded with the nuclear surface.

These were some of the considerations taken into account in this study. To analyze briefly the series presented here, the following considerations may help: 104 males and 107 females were included in the glandular series. A CVS syndrome also occurred in thirty-five males who had a glandular syndrome (37 percent) and in forty-six females (45 percent). Likewise, a similar proportion also had a CNS syndrome. In some, the CVS or CNS lesion proved to be lethal, yet in others, after the CVS or CNS illness abated, the glandular syndrome could persist and in a few went on to malignancy. This was found chiefly to be retroperitoneal and of pancreatic origin. The proportion is shown in Figure 5.3.

The incidence of retroperitoneal malignancy apparently having an origin in the pancreas does appear to be sinister. The sex differences are too small to be statistically significant. Also, it must be noted that more than one gland was affected in some patients, and in some cases both CVS and CNS syndromes were present with a glandular component.

In all of these cases, a minimum of a fourfold rise in circulating enterovirus antibodies, with a positive ELISA IgM and later IgG, was accepted as defining the viral etiology, and in 20 percent a positive culture was also obtained. In the 1980s, when Professor Mowbray's VP1 test was available, it greatly aided in the definition of persisting enteroviral infection. A high or rising ESR performed at the time of illness would arouse suspicion of an acute response to infection or, more likely, the beginning of an autoimmune syndrome with all that that could mean, either at the time of the presenting illness or later. This was discussed in previous paragraphs. Serial titers over months, and in some cases years, were performed. Without these no serious conclusions would be possible. The VP1 test, which is so helpful, was not initially available. As these criteria apply to all the cases, I do not give details of the individual serological tests in each case.

FIBROMYALGIA

Apart from purely glandular effects, muscle pathology may also be a discrete result of virus-induced illness. In the past, this was often disguised under the term "fibrositis," which was often used for conditions of both muscle and extraskeletal tenderness and pain. The

FIGURE 5.3. Analysis of Cases with Glandular Syndromes After Viral Infection

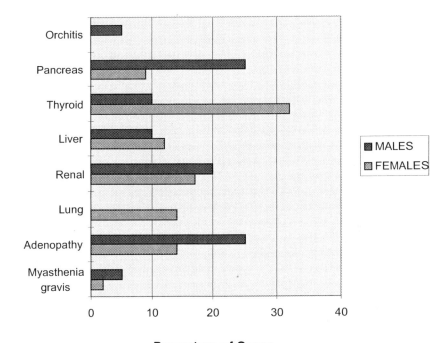

Percentage of Cases

Males: Twenty cases with glandular syndromes from 125 cases who also had a CNS syndrome

Females: Forty-three cases with glandular syndromes from 263 cases who also had a CNS syndrome

term "fibromyalgia" (FM) should be more carefully used to denote a muscle-related painful condition.

Prevalence

Fibromyalgia is diagnosed in about 15 percent of cases seen by a rheumatologist.

Symptoms

Symptoms may vary, and some of them are not directly related to FM but are of the same basic etiology. The symptoms directly due to

FM are in nonarticular structures, chiefly in muscles and tendons and occasionally in bursae, which may be swollen (e.g., Baker's cyst).

Collateral Symptoms

Collateral symptoms include IBS, which occurs in about 40 percent of cases, and insomnia, which is not particularly due to the pain but appears to originate more in the central nervous system. Tingling feelings that are sometimes painful are felt in the limbs. The actual muscle symptoms occur in the neck—often in the trapezius muscle in the chest, where they may be so marked that they resemble angina. Pain in the back and sacral areas, which is also in the muscles of lower limbs, may mimic disc lesions. Naturally, stiffness that makes movement difficult is disconcerting, and the effort to overcome the symptoms by exertion, while at the time appearing beneficial, may leave the patient exhausted later. The next day may be spent in bed as a consequence. This is common and, unfortunately, in some cases when an examining physician requests the patient to do a number of exercises, he or she would have to see the same patient the next day to assess the result of the requested exercise.

Differential Diagnosis

It is not intended to fully explore differential diagnosis, for the symptoms and signs are definite when carefully evaluated. However, the weakness is similar to that of myasthenia gravis, and I have seen four such cases in equal sex proportions. Polymyositis, which is more systemic in distribution, and also rheumatic disorders, should be fairly easily defined. Systemic lupus erythematosus more often affects joint areas and of course has other manifestations ranging from skin to heart and kidneys, often including liver palm and butterfly rash.

The only symptoms that may cause confusion are marked "central" symptoms that include gross sleep disturbance (owl syndrome), gross fatigue that inhibits both physical and mental activity (the latter involving inability to grasp what is heard or read, as well as anomia and short-term memory impairment), and also focusing difficulties and audiosensitivity. The diagnosis would then change from fibromyalgia to myalgic encephalomyelitis. Polymyalgia rheumatica is perhaps more difficult to distinguish, as it involves is pain and stiffness in similar muscle groups but not the same weakness.

Glycogen storage disease and certain myopathies in which muscle metabolism is abnormal are more rare and again more generalized and diffuse.

Physical Examination

In this series one essential finding involves specific "tender points." These are locally very painful, soft to palpation, and do not show any signs of "referred pain." They are fairly common in the shoulder areas, biceps, trapezius, and supraspinatus, and still more common in the lower limbs, and in the calf muscles, where wasting is not unusual. The rectus abdominis is not an infrequent site, and two cases in this series, both males, had to have resultant hernias repaired—one man on two separate occasions. It is essential to distinguish these softened tender areas from the even more obvious tender palpable "nodules" seen in fibrositis or other muscle disorders such as myofacial pain-dysfunction syndrome. These tender areas are only part of the whole muscle pathology, and usually palpation of other areas of the involved muscle is likewise painful.

There is, however, the possibility of a link between muscle disorder and CNS disorder, as seen in poliomyelitis and parkinsonism. Some signs that help to differentiate fibromyalgia are shown in Table 5.2.

TABLE 5.2. Signs to Differentiate a CNS Disorder and a Muscle Disorder

Neurological Origin	Muscle Origin
Wasting +++	Wasting +
Weakness varies	Weakness ++
Reflexes poor	Reflexes normal
• little weakness of response	• weakness of response ++
Sensory changes in affected areas	No sensory changes
• in some cases	

To differentiate between upper and lower motor neuron response may be worthwhile.

Upper Motor Neuron Disease	Lower Motor Neuron Disease
Reflexes +++	Reflexes poor to absent
Atrophy absent	Atrophy present
Fasciculations absent	Fasciculations present
Tone +++	Tone poor to absent

However, some patients may describe the feelings in the muscles as weakness when really it is fatigue, and this may be due to intrinsic muscle abnormality, or central fatigue may be hypothalamically mediated.

Other signs may also be considered in light of the neuromyalgic signs mentioned. Muscle jitter occurs in some cases and may be very obvious. Asking the patient to be seated and then, with a leg outstretched, to raise and lower the foreleg from the knee joint, results in jitter, which I have videotaped.

Cephalalgia

Headache is very common in this group also, and, after excluding sinister pathology such as intracranial lesions, attention should be given to the areas affected, for in anxiety states and conversion hysteria the headaches are nearly always bitemporal. Those in FM syndrome are usually fronto-occipital and relate to muscle tension. Sometimes such headaches are seen apart from FM. Fonto-occipital headaches, therefore, are merely an extension or result of the upper cervical muscle involvement. ESR testing can differentiate between FM and cases in which autoimmune reactions dominate. In true FM the ESR is usually in the normal range.

Pathology

There is a similitarity between pathology in peripheral muscles and in cardiac muscles. Cases cited elsewhere include endocardial fibroeastosis, which results from a proliferation of collagenous and elastic tissue. It can also interfere with the vascular supply to adjacent myocardial muscles. On the other hand, in endomyocardial fibrosis, dense fibrous tissue invades the muscle, but elastic tissue is not apparent. In both conditions, as well as FM, virus has been isolated from the muscle. The mitochondria are usually affected in FM, and intracellular enzymes with or without protein deficiency can be demonstrated. Lactic acid is found in higher than normal concentrations as a result of impaired metabolism. These facts were presented in a meeting at Charing Cross many years ago. On microscopy, some muscle fibers are atrophied. A sample that was biopsied from muscle in a very young man many years ago was said to show only the marked signs of aging. Adipose tissue and fat had replaced the atrophic fibers in this case, and it was significant that his CPK was raised as it has been in many investigated since.

Another case involved a female patient in her thirties (F12) who satisfied the criteria for FM. She had the usual high titers for CBV group 3 and also a positive VP1. A muscle biopsy was performed, with this report:

> Further to my letter of 16 August [1975] this lady had a needle muscle biopsy performed on the 16th September. The biopsy shows scattered fibres with peripheral aggregation of mitochondria in the succinate dehydrogenase preparations. At least some of these fibres have low or absent cytochrome *c* oxidase activity. There can be little doubt that this biopsy is abnormal although only a few fibers are affected. How much of this is actually related to the lady's pain is at present impossible to say. However, she clearly requires further investigation and, in view of this, I am arranging for her to be exorcised [exercised??] on the 8th November and will let you know the results in due course.

Electron microscopy has shown an organism similar to picornavirus in some of these cases and also in polymyositis and dermatomyositis. In some cases coxsackie A9 as well as the B group have been isolated.

Cofactors are relevant, and no doubt many variants will appear. Cofactors may be as diverse as a deficiency of host chemical factors, such as enzymes or specific inorganic elements, or the additive effects of extraneous elements such as insecticides and organisms such as viruses. The prions have been shown to cause bovine spongiform encephalopathy in cattle as well as many diseases in humans. The effects of a deficiency of host chemical factors have been demonstrated in selenium deficiency. This selenium deficiency resulted in alterations in certain genomic strands in Coxsackievirus-infected mice. In both cases, the effects on the prion or viral particle rendered it virulent to the brain or myocardium. This virulence, which depended upon viral strand change in the selenium-deficient host, persisted when another host was infected with the virus.

From my own work I suggest the following questions and tentative answers:

1. Why, in poliomyelitis, does exercise so markedly result in severe paralysis in the early stages?

> From research it is obvious that virus infects muscle cells. It can proliferate in muscle fibers and then, reaching the motor endplate, the virus has access to the neuron supplying that fiber. From there the cerebrospinal fluid becomes infected and, as in herpes zoster, there is a channel for virus activity back to the spinal cord—in the case of herpes to the posterior cord cells, and in poliomyelitis to the anterior horn cells. Exercising an affected muscle exacerbates this process by increasing the turnover of virus and its passage into the CSF. This was apparent in my own early practice and sadly occurred in a member of my family who, by rowing for a college regatta, developed polio paralysis of the chest respiratory musculature and later polioencephalitis and died. I postulated then, and do so now, that the virus entered the brain, resulting in infection, via the spinal fluid.

2. Why, in the case of herpes zoster, are only the cells of the posterior horn affected, while poliomyelitis affects only the cells of the anterior horn, even though they are anatomically so close and subject to the same CSF circulation?

> That these two structures are not simultaneously affected is shown by the pain without paralysis in the former and paralysis without pain in the latter. The reason may be that viral transport is confined by the periaxonal sheath. However, access to CSF, and its possible implication in viral transport, has to be considered. This may raise a question about the specificity of end organ receptors in these cells—in one case for the herpes zoster virus and in the other for poliovirus. That this mechanism may not always be strictly specific is evidenced by the infection of other CNS tissue by the poliovirus, as in posterior and bulbar poliomyelitis and encephalitis. This may be due to genomic mutation within the viral strands, which thus eludes the specificity of the receptors and allows more generalized access to other cells in the CNS.

3. What is the difference—if any—between "central fatigue" and peripheral or muscle fatigue?

In this series, over the decades it was obvious that the two were quite distinct, for cognitive processes were involved as well as other modalities of sensation. From the previous answer it is obvious that there is a continuum between the CFS of the spinal cord and the brain and this involves any viral activity, the midbrain being the first location to be affected. This organic diversity involves the hypothalamus, as shown elsewhere, including the reticulum cell formation through which afferent sensations are relayed, monitored, and then, where appropriate, transferred to the higher centers. This is dealt with in Chapter 3. However, it is worthwhile to mention again that SPET scans show hypoperfusion in these areas, which validates the observation that this subtentorial, midbrain area is perhaps more susceptible to infection.

Muscle fatigue, however, has been shown to be due to abnormal metabolic changes, as mentioned earlier.

EXAMPLES

Pancreas

- Males; there were fifteen out of the 104 glandular cases (14.4 percent) and two of these eventually became malignant. Ten developed diabetes (9.6 percent).
- Females; there were seventeen out of 107 (15.8 percent), and one of these developed a malignancy. Fourteen also became diabetic (13 percent).

The percentage of females with diabetes in those with pancreatic syndromes was a little higher than that for males in this series; this may suggest that the female is more vulnerable, but further work is required to establish this.

Thyroid Antibodies

Among males, only two developed antibodies (only 2 percent) and one developed myxoedema later. However, for females, twenty-two developed antibodies (20.5 percent). Three of these developed myxedema (2.8 percent). This shows the female predominance in this section for the development of thyroid antibodies, but, surprisingly enough, the development of antibodies did not correlate well with the development of overt thyroid failure.

It is significant however that, though both sexes developed antibodies, the rate of actual thyroid failure for those who did develop antibodies was 0.9 percent for males and 2.8 percent for females. Thus, females appear to be seven times more prone to hypothyroidism in this series.

Liver

In the male series, nine developed hepatic symptoms (8.6 percent). They had abnormal liver function tests, but not due to Hepatitis A, B, or C.

In the female series, seven developed hepatic symptoms (6.5 percent). They also had abnormal liver function tests, again, not due to hepatitis virus A, B, or C. Two females had needle biopsies, which demonstrated a vasculitis of the liver. In this case as in others, well-marked liver palm was sometimes in evidence and photographed at the time of illness. These signs remitted when recovery occurred.

Kidney

Among males, seven developed renal pathology (7.4 percent). Three were acute and remitted. Four developed hypertension and one eventually required dialysis. This young man also had myocarditis. A biopsy of the kidney at the time demonstrated vasculitis, but not glomerulitis. Unfortunately, a suitable donor was not found, but he was found dead in bed years later from the cardiac effects of his illness.

Among females, seven developed renal pathology (6.5 percent). Four were acute and remitted. Three developed hypertension, and one of these required dialysis. She eventually had a renal transplant. She remains satisfactory at this writing.

In this series the biopsies showed glomerulitis with sparing of the actual nephron. The outcome appeared to be the same in both sexes. Some made a good recovery after the initial acute illness, but this took months. Those who progressed to the chronic stage did not do well, as shown earlier.

Stomach and Bowel (Acute Gastritis and/or Colitis or IBS)

Nine males had stomach and bowel problems (8.6 percent). These cases are worth noting, as three had the typical initial phlegmonous type of viral gastritis, which remitted. Petechial hemorrhages in this type of case can be seen in the posterior pharynx if carefully examined. These extend down the esophagus to the stomach. The vomit has a gravylike consistency and contains frank or occult blood. This occurred in one nine-year-old boy and was so severe in the first few days that he had to be admitted to the hospital and transfused. He made a good recovery without sequelae. A forty-year-old man in 1980 had a severe attack, collapsed, and was admitted to the hospital. He too required transfusion, and eventually a partial gastrectomy was performed to arrest the ongoing hemorrhage. He went on to hepatorenal failure and was in the intensive care unit for a while, but recovered and is now quite well. His serial titers were high, as in the others, and in his case also a positive culture was obtained. He is mentioned as his daughter also became ill with the same viral strain and had severe anorexia, from which she also eventually made a good recovery.

Another case, M25, who was fifty-eight years of age, had a similar illness. I saw him with viral gastroenteritis, which continued with rather chronic gastric discomfort. I referred him for endoscopy, and he was gastroscoped, but no ulcer was found. Approximately ten to fourteen days later he collapsed. I was called and had him admitted immediately. Unfortunately, about twelve hours later he died due to a large bleeding ulcer that had eroded the right gastric artery, as shown in Figure 5.4.

We discussed the case later, but it was still confirmed that the earlier endoscopy did not reveal an ulcer. It is my contention that this can occur, and as in a varicose ulcer, the initial lesion is beneath the gastric mucosa, which later breaks down with quite extensive ulceration and in this case, severe hemorrhage.

A further case in 1978 was M26, a sixty-year-old man who had viral myocarditis and later a clinical esophagitis and gross anemia. His hemoglobin was only 5.6. Coxsackie B group 4 titers rose to 1/512, and his complement CH50 fell to 26 percent and C3 to 56 percent—he had a positive IgM and IgG later. He was admitted and investigated, and nothing malignant was found. His illness remitted, and for several years he seemed reasonably well. He then began to have some chest discomfort, and renewed investigation showed a diffuse, spreading mediastinal neoplasm of presumed esophageal origin, from which he died.

In another case referred to in the CVS series (Family 07), after an initial viral myocarditis, a man developed subacute abdominal pain and was operated on for appendicitis. A carcinoma of the tip of the appendix was found on histology. He did not have any sequelae to this, but years later he had a pancreatitis, as shown elsewhere in this series, and died years after from a carcinoma of the pancreas. His wife had an absolutely identical illness with the same sequelae and is also referred to.

Other cases developed severe irritable bowel syndromes. This syndrome occurred in about 10 percent of both male and female cases, as discussed later. In my experience this is not unusual, as is the occurrence of food and alcohol intolerance. The latter can greatly exacerbate both gastric and pancreatic symptoms. It is interesting, as noted in Chapter 3, that the hypothalamus has a profound effect on bowel activity. In animals it has been found that a dysfunction of alveolar macrophages in the Peyer's patches is linked with a rise in monilial colony formation. These macrophages, in a virus-infected mouse

FIGURE 5.4. Bleeding Ulcer Causing Erosion of Right Gastric Artery

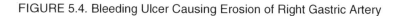
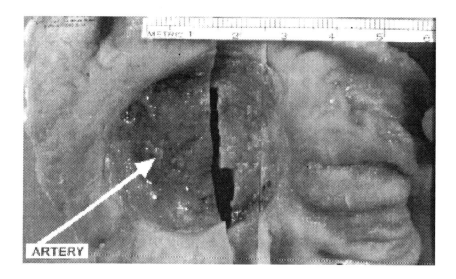

model, fail to digest minute instilled latex particles, which are usually digested by normal macrophages (Loria, 1986a). The result is that in the healthy animal only 20 percent of the ingested latex particles are excreted as the rest are absorbed by the macrophages, but in the infected animal 80 percent are excreted and recovered. This article discusses immunosuppression in animals and is very helpful. To extrapolate, it would appear reasonable to assume that the apparent increase in monilia in these cases is also the result of the inactivity of the macrophages in the Peyer's patches of the bowel.

Among females, seven cases are reported here (6.5. percent). These were also acute phlegmonous gastritis and/or colitis or IBS. One of these remitted, and one went on to have IBS. One developed a type of ileocolitis with fistula formation. My friend and colleague Dr. T. H. Tweedy, FRCS, operated on her, and histology showed large numbers of plasma cells, but we were never able to define whether this was a type of Crohn's disease or ulcerative colitis. It carried the signs of both. Sadly, she lost a great deal of weight and died in her forties, but without ensuing malignancy. I had thought of obtaining some thalidomide for her, but we were too late. A similiar case (published in the *BMJ*) occurred in a doctor working in leprosy who was conversant with the use of thalidomide. She treated herself with thalidomide and had a very good remission. Thalidomide has been shown to have a suppressive autoimmune reaction and to be useful in nodular leprosy and of course is still being used.

Another female, F32, had an odd sequel to enteroviral infection. Her cecum was affected, and she had intermittent swelling in the RIF which would occur spontaneously. On palpation, it appeared to be about the size of a melon, and she was very uncomfortable. Again, Dr. T. H. Tweedy operated on her and I assisted, and on opening the abdomen the cecum did indeed balloon to the size of a melon. This was resected and the ileum anastomosed to the upper ascending colon. On histology the circular muscle was seen to be grossly atrophied, thus allowing the balloon-like distension, which could be palpated. Later she had an anal prolapse of the sigmoid colon, which Dr. Tweedy repaired. He buttressed the omentum to prevent further prolapse. This case is significant, as enteroviruses have been recovered from the muscle cells of bowel.

The daughter of the male patient who had the partial gastrectomy, alluded to earlier, developed a similar illness at the same time as her father, with similar titers. She developed severe anorexia and lost a great deal of weight but recovered. Conversely, in 1991, another female patient had a gastric viral illness and subsequently developed bulimia. Both these cases were quite severe and lasted for many months after the initial viral illness. Some would consider them a psychiatric consequence of the primary illness, but it is my opinion that they were both mediated by a consequent hypothalamic dysfunction.

Two cases of particular interest occurred in 1978 and 1979. They were somewhat similar to the two cases described in the previous paragraph. Because of my research interest in apparent coxsackie-mediated diseases, I was asked to attend a clinical postgraduate meeting where a case was presented of a woman who had had intense abdominal pain during the last trimester of pregnancy. Like the one described in another chapter (the mother of case M20), it was thought she might have an abruptioplacentea, but it was not. However, the baby died in utero. After delivery she still had the pain, and eventually a total colectomy was performed, as it was thought that *Clostridium welchii* had been recovered from her stools. This was later shown to be incorrect. Subsequent histology only showed the muscular coats of the colon to be heavily congested with plasma cells, and no infarct or other pathology was found.

At about the same time I was asked to see a woman of similar age and, suspecting an appendicitis, visited her home. On examination, I came to the conclusion that she had a severe Bornholm type of pain similar to the previous case. She was admitted to the hospital, where she came under the care of Dr. D. Chadwick, who at the time was senior registrar. We found that bowel sounds were absent, but no other pathological signs were found. She was treated for acute coxsackie enterocolitis and was parentally fed by IV drip and had gastric suction for some weeks. This case was later presented by Dr. Chadwick at a postgraduate meeting, as it was assumed her recovery was complete. However, months later it became apparent that she had some residual mass in the RIF. My surgical colleague, R. Bearne, FRCS, operated on her, and she was found to have a very inflamed ileocecal area with omentum adherent. The appendix, which was normal, was removed, and she made a good recovery. Her illness was identical to the aforementioned case except that she was not pregnant. Fortunately for her we saved her colon.

It may be appropriate to mention the outcome of several who have had laparoscopies. We have found and aspirated straw-colored fluid, and in one a mass of adhesions was also found. One of these patients, whose titers were high with an ELISA IgM positive test, later became pregnant. I delivered the baby (case F33) and watched her very carefully afterward. Later heart murmurs developed, and she required open heart surgery for the congenital defects. In this case there was a strong family history of viral illness, as mentioned in Chapter 4.

It is also interesting that during 1978, the side effects of practolol were much in the public eye as a cause of retroperitoneal fibrosis. On gathering as many papers as possible and analyzing them, it was apparent that this particular beta-blocker had been used in cases where dysrythmias were a problem. As seen in Chapter 2, this type of dysrythmia occurred fairly often with viral myocarditis. However, no mention was made of the cause of the dysrythmias in the reports, but it is a tantalizing thought that maybe they were of viral origin. If so, then maybe, as with others in this series, the retroperitoneal fibrosis could be of viral etiology also. No proof either way was given and the matter remains sub judice.

Lungs

Both males and females in equal proportions presented with viral pneumonitis demonstrated by X ray, which remitted. In other cases other sequelae occurred, or later progressed to quite severe stenosing alveolitis, with fatal results. Mediastinitis and also pleurisy can follow viral infections, and the former may give rise to a pericardial friction rub without the heart being affected, while the latter may give rise to a pleural friction rub without the lungs being affected. There were eleven males and eleven females.

One interesting case in the series relating to pulmonary infections occurred in a young female (Family 09) who previously had had many serial virological titers performed, all of which were positive for enteroviral infection as in the rest of this series. She developed a mass in the chest, demonstrated on X ray, which had not been present on prior occasions. It was removed and proved to be a large retropleural dermoid cyst. Previous X rays, years earlier, had not shown any mass. It is again my view that viral stimulation to the rudimentary line of cells, which must have been there since birth, resulted in the development of this dermoid cyst, which measured $10 \times 5 \times 4$ cm. Later she developed severe ME with all the usual symptoms, and later still she developed mycosis fungoides, which happily remitted. Her history is included in Chapter 3 in more detail. At this writing, her recovery has been good following IgG therapy.

Thymus

In this series, one male seventeen years of age and an older man in his fifties, as well as one female in her twenties and another in her fifties, developed myasthenia gravis after an initial coxsackie B viral illness . This also is discussed in more detail in Chapter 5 and is evidence of the household function of the cell being impaired without actual cell death. The glandular dysfunctions that may be hypothalamically mediated are also discussed in Chapter 3 and have been omitted here. However, it may be relevant to repeat that some syndromes apparently due to glandular dysfunction may actually be due to the failure of that particular gland to produce its secretions. As shown in Chapter 3, it is also possible that more central lack of control and stimulation of the gland in question may be the cause of the dysfunction.

Finally, it should be apparent that a single glandular dysfunction may have multiple effects through a synergism with other glands or organs. Examples could be cited, such as hypothyroidism resulting in a myxedematous heart, or thymic dysfunction resulting in the muscle weakness of myasthenia gravis, or the pancreas and diabetes, as well as the menstrual cycle dysfunction or acromegally that may result from pituitary changes. Each one of these has been noted and carefully documented in this series (see Table 5.3). It is not suggested that a viral infection is the only cause of the syndromes outlined here, but these cases are examples of many more that were carefully assessed and in which the viral etiology was convincingly defined. Teratogenic and carcinogenic effects are omitted but are discussed in the appropriate chapters.

This is an analysis of all the syndromes, and more than one syndrome of the same autoimmune etiology occurred in a rare case. Although the glandular syndrome itself was most significant in some, in others, while perhaps persisting, it was not the chief cause of the patient's general debility, which in some cases was ME or myocarditis. Two of the latter received heart transplants. However, one

TABLE 5.3. Statistical Summary of Case Reports

	Males		Females	
	Number	**Percentage**	**Number**	**Percentage**
Pancreas	15	14.4	17	15.8
Diabetes	10	9.6	14	13.0
Thyroid	2	2.0	22	20.5
Myxedema	1	0.9	3	2.8
Liver	9	8.6	7	6.5
Lung	11	10.5	11	10.2
Adenopathy	26	25.0	18	16.8
Gonads	3	2.9	6	5.6
Appendix	2	2.0	3	2.8
Gastric	9	8.6	7	6.8
Renal	7	7.4	7	6.5
Thymus	2	2.0	2	1.8
Total Cases	**97**		**117**	
Total Syndromes	**104**		**107**	

of the males and one female had severe renal disease. The female had a kidney transplant, but the young man died of myocarditis before one could be performed.

Other odd syndromes as diverse as Sjögren's syndrome and asthma also occurred and are recorded. They are not detailed here but could possibly be an outcome of the original viral infection. In this series, more specific glandular syndromes are detailed. It is interesting that the computerized records shown in Table 5.3 yield a total of 97 "primary" syndromes in the 104 in the male series, which is 93 percent, and an even higher percentage in the 107 in the female series. Thus, to illustrate, there were only nineteen male ME cases in the glandular series (18 percent), whereas there were thirty-nine females (36 percent). Thirty-four males had coexisting cardiovascular consequences (32.6 percent), and forty-two females (39 percent).

Clinically it must be emphasized that while these syndromes coexist and should be sought and then related to a common etiology if appropriate, it is not always apparent which single syndrome is the main cause of the patient's debility.

Chapter 6

Host Factors in Viruses and Toxins

One theory I would like to challenge is reflected in statements such as, "Oh, it is just a virus" or "bacteria" or "toxin," for the host has an effect on any absorbed material, and obviously the reverse is true. So the absorption, distribution, metabolism, and excretion of xenobiotics are host factors. Once absorbed, substances such as viruses, xenobiotics, antibiotics, or even food have an interaction with host cells, maybe at intracellular levels, or with the structural proteins of the capsule, which would have effects on enzyme or receptor activity. A chain response may follow, the character of which will depend on the function of the organ that has suffered, e.g., if the kidney or the lung is damaged then excretion or respiration change occurs.

This is obvious as a theory, but the multiplicity of etiological factors that may produce a similar effect is not by any means always obvious, much less reckoned with. The effects of these varying elements in the environment on the host may produce pathological effects, but we should also consider that the host itself changes these elements for its own good, or occasionally to its own detriment, and in some cases a substance cannot be detoxified and is harmful in itself. The first case can be illustrated by the action of the host on wholesome food, which is absorbed for good. Moreover, the gut bacteria *(E. coli),* acting in symbiosis, partake of such food, and in return their "excreta" from the cell membrane give us some of our vitamin B supply. Conversely, those same bacteria may convert innocuous substances into carcinogens (e.g., cycasin into methylazoxymethanol). On the other hand, the host itself may break down a substance into less toxic metabolites.

Another factor is the rate of excretion of a foreign substance, and this may be of paramount importance, especially if the host is being exposed at intervals to additive amounts which may accumulate. This would apply to drugs given for therapeutic reasons and also to toxins to which we may be inadvertently exposed. A good example here is the cardiovascular drug amiodarone, which though slowly absorbed is bound to plasma proteins, and its half-life can be sixty days. Though the desired effect is on the heart, its concentration is greater in other tissues (e.g., lungs, liver, eyes, and thyroid). Thus the word "side effects" is a misnomer, for it generates the idea that these are less potent than the desired target effect, whereas they can be harmful, out of proportion to any beneficial effect, as with other drugs or toxins.

Lastly, a substance may have different effects over time, e.g., it may be hepatotoxic in an acute dose or carcinogenic in repeated small doses. It is a sine que non that the minimum lethal dose (MLD) applies to the first kind of effect but has no meaning as far as long-term insidious effects are concerned. Furthermore, as shown previously, the action observed in one organ (e.g., liver or heart) may not be the lethal factor, which may be toxicity in another organ (e.g., the CNS). This is illustrated above in the case of amiodarone.

Another serious consideration is the difference between reversible and nonreversible reactions, which may lie in the type of tissue affected. If a reaction occurs in a receptor where "release" is possible, no further harm might be expected, and the reaction is reversible (e.g., beta-blockers). If, however, nuclear DNA was affected, then tumor growth may occur years later and the initiating factor may not be detected. Not only can this occur with inorganic compounds, but in this series the "sick cell syndrome" generated by viral infection can be the precursor of malignancy, and again the time involved may well mask the etiological factor. The cell membrane itself has not been given enough attention and is often considered merely as containing the important intracellular mitochondria, DNA, etc. It fulfills the functioning role of the cell, however, either, as in the CNS, by transmitting impulses, or, as in the thymus, adrenal, thyroid, or pancreas, by the secretion of enzymes. These functions can all be shown to be affected by toxins and viruses, for example, as in diabetes or myasthenia gravis.

Thus, we have to consider anything that may point to membrane dysfunction. Some workers have stressed essential fatty acids (EFA), and the consequential changes which may occur point to cell membrane dysfunction (Winther, 1991). The question to consider here is whether this dysfunction is mediated by the EFAs per se, whether the changes in the EFAs are due to viral insult and the membrane dysfunction is a sequel. I believe that it may be either or both. In certain genetic strains there may be primary dysfunction at the level of gammalinolenc acid, while in others membrane dysfunction may be impaired by viral infection. Thus many functional changes may occur, from the mitochondria to the EFAs of the membrane. There is no suggestion that the mitochondria initiate the malady, and I suggest that EFAs do not do so either. This does not mean that a subject with a membrane dysfunction would not be more susceptible. I have found in many cases a well-defined change in sensitivity that could be a result of this. Thus, the role of membrane activity may be looked at as mediatorial.

Likewise, we may ask whether EFAs are mediators for the production of receptors, etc., on the cell membrane or for the function of the receptors and enzymes, as in syndromes already noted. The prostaglandins and leukotrienes are also EFA-dependent products. Thus it would appear that interferon exerts its effect through the cyclooxygenase enzyme, and if this is absent, as in some genetic defects, then there is a lack of antiviral activity. What might be considered inactivity on the part of interferons is actually due to deficiency of the substrate through which the IFN exerts its antiviral activity.

As postulated elsewhere, the gut is the most complex organ for autoimmune and antigen processing and is referred to by Galland (Jenkins and Mowbray, 1991). This should be considered by some who claim that bowel organisms (monilia) are "causal" in the ME syndrome when an identical reasoning could be to indicate that the imbalance is due to macrophage inability to phagocytose thrush organisms, and that this inability is due to the viral infection rather than a cause of it.

METABOLISM

The creation of metabolites from parent compounds may produce a toxic substance as well as facilitate the elimination of the compound.

Lipid-soluble compounds are perhaps poorly metabolized and may have half-lives of months or years. They may facilitate the transport of both viruses and inorganic toxins and can pass the blood-brain barrier and hence be a CNS hazard.

Metabolism may be affected by the following:

1. *Oxidation* occurs by the microsomal monooxygenase system of the endoplasmic reticulum of cells in the tissues, particularly the liver and the Clara cells of the lung. The enzyme is cytochrome oxidase. This process is constant and part of general metabolism, as seen in the monamine oxidases in the CNS. However, an excess of free oxygen radicals may in some cases be harmful, and to a certain extent the host is protected by alpha-tocopherol (Vitamin E).
2. *Reduction.* In some cases it can render a substance water soluble and thus enable renal excretion. Vitamin C is useful.
3. *Hydrolysis.* This relates to reduction also, for some lipids may be rendered water soluble as are inorganic elements (e.g., salts etc.).

Humans are able to carry out most of the metabolic transformations found in other mammals and do not show any significant difference in the enzymatic pathways involved. Thus, though they are all very complex, for our purpose we can say that what affects our living environment will also affect us for good or ill.

Internally, there are host factors that may modify normal metabolism. One example is genetic variants, such as Gilbert's syndrome, with reduced glucuronosyltransferase, which normally conjugates bilirubin. This renders the host cells susceptible to certain drugs that compete for it and may result in high levels of unconjugated bilirubin with resulting jaundice and, if severe, brain damage.

Racial differences also exist. For instance, Egyptians have slow acetylation while the Japanese are fast.

Chronic exposure to some autoimmune inducing or inhibiting agents may be the main factor in the development of a toxic response to another compound or even virus. This is what we may call a cofactor and may not be recognized. It may be in the diet, perhaps the preservatives, pesticides, or food additives.

Any attack on nucleic acid could theoretically result in the host producing an abnormal fetus, or result in a carcinoma in an adult. Examples have been cited and include drugs, toxins, and viruses. Drugs may be exemplified by thalidomide or, more recently, by the use of the drug diphenylhydantoin. A case in recent years involved a severely epileptic young mother, who was taking this drug and did not consult a doctor prior to conception. She was first seen when she was about twelve weeks pregnant. The baby has the hallmarks of drug teratogenicity, particularly the tiny fingernails and small facial features. Smoking as a causal factor for underweight babies, as well as carcinoma, should be well known and is another example of an inorganic medium. I have recognized low folate levels for more than three decades, but for two decades low levels have been shown to occur as a sequel to acute viral infections and constitute a teratogenic hazard.

After four decades of study of the host effects of viruses and toxins, it is obvious that our facilities for defining the etiological agent in illness is very imprecise. It can be shown that only a fourfold recent rise in viral titer may be significant, whereas a high titer of perhaps 1/512 may be present for a year or more in a patient who has largely recovered. This could be construed as the immune system being highly active in the second case and not so efficient in the former.

What remains uncertain is the cofactors, for the family studies show that where one member has succumbed to a virus, other members can have equally high serological titers and no illness. If it was possible to do extensive serological examinations for immune responses in every case and examine all the lymphocyte subsets, look at serological levels of varying toxins, and do tests such as the VP1, then we might perhaps be more likely to define the varying risk cofactors. It is interesting that in animals the alveolar macrophage activity of the gut can be measured by studying how much *Candida albicans* or latex particles are excreted. The assumption might be made that the excess of *Candida* is the real source of illness, whereas it is really a reflection of macrophage incompetence.

Similarly, one virus may well be the trigger for serendipitous invasion by another, more potent virus or even bacteria. This can be seen in AIDS with the invasion of *Pneumocystis carinii* and after varying immunization programs that have resulted in cases of encephalitis which were not due directly to the inoculated agent, but perhaps to the stimulation of a latent virus. Cytomegalovirus (CMV) is such a serendipitous invader and is more frequently seen as a mark of immunosuppression, either by medical management after transplant or sometimes as a result of another viral infection or toxins. Although it is not usually lethal in adults, recently a thirty-one-year-old male patient died suddenly from myocarditis, and at the end of extensive tests the likely agent appears to be CMV. CMV can and does affect pregnant females and has had severe results for the fetus.

A recent example involved a man with ME. He had high levels of CMV antibodies, and I might have passed this over had not his wife alerted me to the fact that their daughter, who was positive for CMV, had just had a full-term stillborn baby and the stillbirth was attributed to this organism.

One thing that viruses have in common with any other toxic agent is the production of idiotypic or autoantibodies. It can be shown that anything that alters the cell membrane expression of "self"—be it virus or toxin—may initiate this mimicry. There are tissues in the body that normally are not vascularized and the lymphocytes never scan, including the cornea, brain, and certain collagen tissues. Should these be damaged by toxin, viral insult, an accident, or even the surgeon's knife, then vascularization may take place and lymphocyte scanning, maybe for the first time, treats the tissue as foreign and produces antibodies. This occurs in certain cases of rheumatoid arthritis and sympathetic opthalmia. The result can be widespread autoimmune attack on similar tissue in other organs. Conversely, scanning by lymphocytes can be inhibited, which occurs when tissue is coated by such protective substances as HCG.

In pregnancy this inhibition is desirable and prevents NK cell activity from destroying the fetus. However, in cases of carcinoma, where the sick cell becomes "embryogenic," it may be treated as a "fetal cell" and coated with HCG. One case had hepatic secondaries on MRI scanning, and the histological report on the primary adenocarcinoma of the gut stated that there was no lymphoid response to be seen. A pregnancy test for HCG on the patient's urine was positive, and the patient was a male (see Figure 6.1).

Summing up, therefore, we can say we have evidence for varying types of cellular insult at target organ levels and also immune dysfunction, but broadly speaking this can be categorized as "suppression" or "enhancement." While all should be functioning in harmony, andy change either way may have harmful or beneficial effects.

FIGURE 6.1. Urine Analysis for HCG in Cancer

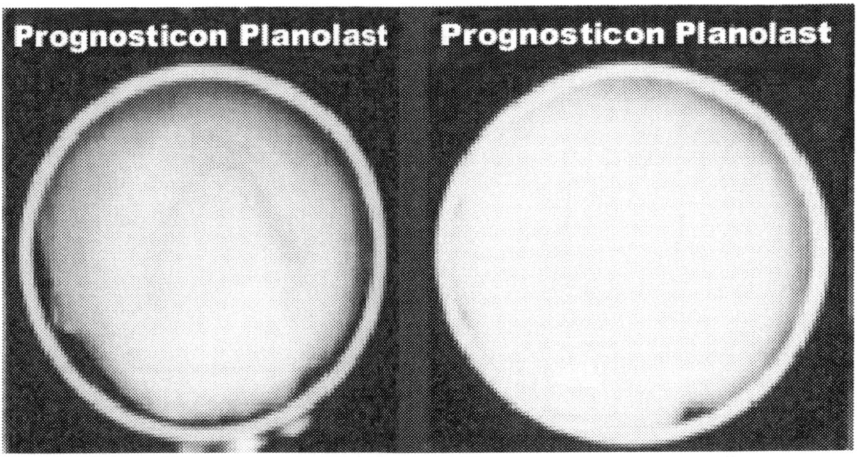

CMV is known to occur in the neonatal period even when the mother is "immune." This has been clearly shown to be due to reactivation of endogenous virus. The virus can be found in urine, saliva, semen, and breast milk. Hence, it can be transmitted either by semen to a partner or breast milk to an infant. Viral shedding can occur years after the initial infection. This brings up the question of host response yet again, and in children the lack of antibodies is most likely the determining factor. This may be modified by acquired genetic predisposition or by mutation of the virus by the mother to be more acceptable to a host of similar genetic disposition, in this instance, the child. However, 90 percent of neonates are clear of disease in these cases, which compares well with only 80 percent for Coxsackievirus infection in the family studies.

Many viruses are known to have teratogenic as well as carcinogenic effects, and the two are not dissimilar. These viruses include the well-known rubella virus, as well as Coxsackievirus. Indeed, in this series the enteroviruses, including ECHO strains, have probably caused more harm than rubella. Kaposi's sarcoma with HIV and Burkitt's lymphoma as well as the occasional oropharyngeal carcinoma following Epstein-Barr virus, together with the late advent of herpes zoster following herpes infection and subacute sclerosing panencephalitis due to latent measles virus, all indicate that persistent viral infection is a reality. It may well be that a similar or a different virus reactivates the dormant offender. This is probably by antigenic drift from the invader to another dormant virus.

NEONATAL ANOMALIES IN VIRAL INFECTIONS

Neonatal anomalies include CNS defects, hepatosplenomegaly, petechiae, retarded growth due to lack of growth hormone, and cardiac defects. In Chapter 4, an overall 30 percent fetal abnormality rate occurred in certain high-risk cases where there was evidence of persisting viral infection.

In the case of CMV, laboratory tests may show thrombocytopenia, high IgM, or conjugated hyperbilirubinemia, as well as an elevated aspartate aminotransferase (AST). These may also be seen in enteroviral infections.

Late signs chiefly seen as a result of CMV infection include the following:

Microcephally	70 percent
Intellectual impairment	60 percent
Neuromuscular disorders	30 percent
Hearing loss	30 percent
Retinitis	22 percent

Moreover, CMV may occasionally lead to cytomegalic inclusion disease, which is associated with an impaired immune syndrome. Intranuclear inclusions are found in enlarged infected cells. Again, the common denominator is a deficiency of immune IgG formation with a lack of cellular immunity.

The condition, as with Coxsackievirus, can manifest itself by interstitial pneumonitis, or areas of gastrointestinal ulceration, or as hepatitis. However, salivary glands may appear to have an adenovirus infection—though CMV is closely related to the herpetic group. In addition, the adrenals, kidney, thyroid, and myocardium may be affected. These conditions may also occur as a result of Coxsackievirus infection.

It has been shown that the day of slow, persistent, or latent viruses has arrived (Melnick, 1974). All-or-none concepts of immunologically mediated viral disease are obsolete, for the diseases studied show various combinations of replicating virus as well as varying levels of cellular immunity. It is possible to have high tissue titers without viremia or antibody (as in scrapie). Other diseases produce high levels of antibodies and elusive but persistent free virus, as in Aleutian mink disease. In humans we have evidence of Coxsackievirus persisting in lymphoid lines, the herpes group persisting in CNS tissue, and CMV persistence. There is clear-cut evidence of the possibility of transmission of the virion of spongiform encephalopathy from animal tissue to humans. The latent period between infection and overt illness, culminating in death from AIDS, should be more than sufficient to cause the medical profession to think more deeply about the longterm effects of virus-mediated illness.

In these studies, the difficulty is compounded by various factors in trying to define the precise etiological agent. Is it one agent—a virus? Is it multiple agents? If so, is it multiple viruses or virus plus an inorganic factor? Is it a slow virus with possible long-term end results and perhaps low serological evidence of its presence (e.g., CMV)? Is it a latent virus that has been activated by some other virus or agent, maybe with raised serological titers (e.g., herpes or coxsackie)? These are all factors to consider in trying to interpret laboratory tests.

However, this may lead us to think in terms of harnessing host factors in treatment of both cancer and virus-induced illness. As an illustration, the advent of the experimental drug Ampligen is worth considering. Basically, it is a mismatched double stranded RNA (ds-RNA) and has been used in HIV cases. It acts as a biotrigger to cause release of lymphokines, as well as being an intracellular cofactor for enzymes of the natural antiviral pathways. Its mismatched region of uracil residues is simply inserted into the polypyrimidine strand, which accelerates ds-RNA hydrolysis and prevents toxicity and replication. It also enhances the antiviral effect of zidovudine and has greater effect than the interferons—the latter act by preventing the decoating of virus, which in turn prevents the replication of its RNA. However, it is uncertain whether a treatment with Ampligen will, for various reasons, gain credence and become readily available.

A more simple and much less potent mechanism was promoted in the 1920s by Professor Coley and involved the injection of *Propionibacterium acnes,* which in turn stimulated the whole immune system and in some cases caused a remission in cancer patients. He had noted cases in which, in a patient with cancer, an intervening illness of bacterial origin sometimes resulted in remission. I have used intraperitoneal infusions of *Propionibacterium acnes* in a number of cases of cancer where there were peritoneal effusions. There were encouraging remissions but, unhappily, no complete cures.

Many years ago, an elderly lady with cancer of the gallbladder, proven at operation, developed severe lobar pneumonia. I said, "We will leave this alone, as it is sometimes called the old folks' friend and gently terminates suffering." She became extremely dehydrated and comatose, but on the tenth day had the typical "crisis" and awakened, and through parched lips asked what day it was. She was fed with sips of water for days to rehydrate her, and she recovered. Several weeks later, when I palpated the abdomen, there was no palpable mass to be found. She lived to attend the funeral of her son, to whose home she had been sent to die. This case confirms the mechanisms involved behind Professor Coley's hypothesis. Had I given her antibiotics for her lobar pneumonia, the beneficial resultant immune reaction that led to the lysis of the cancer cells may not have occurred.

This method of treatment has met with varying degrees of success. At this writing, various colleagues at home and abroad are exploring other host factors. These include thymic humoral factor-$\gamma 2$ (THF-$\gamma 2$), which is an immunomodulatory peptide, as well as melatonin (MLT). Melatonin itself had no effect on virus growth but did appear to increase host resistance to the virus, and it has been reported to stimulate the release of interferon alpha (Ben-Nathan et al., 1995). Other host factors, such as lipids, have been investigated and reported on by various workers, including Professor Roger Loria. The question of the ability of these factors to facilitate the passage of viruses through the blood-brain barrier is intriguing.

Fleischmann described interferons as follows:

> Interferons are cellular proteins which have antiviral, immuno-regulatory, hormonal and anti-proliferative activities [for review, see Baron et al. 1982]. Three types of interferons have been described for both the mouse and human systems; they have been designated interferon alpha (IFN-α), interferon beta (IFN-β) and interferon gamma (IFN-γ). They are differentiated

by their physical and biological properties, by their inducers, and by the cell type in which they are produced. IFN-α and IFN-β appear to be distantly related, while IFN-γ is quite distinct.

It is the immunoregulatory and antiproliferative activities of the interferons which form the basis for the possible use of interferons as anticancer agents.

He published a summary of his work as follows:

The interactions of three types of interferons (IFN-α, IFN-β and IFN-γ) are described. IFN-α combined with IFN-β has an additive effect, but IFN-γ combined with either IFN-α or IFN-β (combination interferon treatment) has a synergistic or potentiating effect originally described in the mouse system as the synergistic enhancement of interferon's antiviral activity. Subsequent studies have shown the potentiation of interferon's NK cell activation, direct antiproliferative activity, and in vivo antitumour activity. Potentiation was readily quantified in the antiproliferative studies and was shown to cause more than 200-fold enhancement or the interferon activity. In vitro studies have shown that potentiation occurs similarly in mouse and human systems. The relative effectiveness of combination interferon treatment was determined on paired sets of nonmalignant and malignant murine cells. Combination interferon treatment had only a slight effect on the nonmalignant cells, but the malignant cells were dramatically slowed in their growth or even killed. Combination treatments with interferon and hyperthermia have shown synergistic interactions, most strongly with IFN-γ with enhancing effects as high as 14-fold. Hyperthermia and interferon, especially IFN-γ and combination interferon treatment, may have particular promise as a cancer therapy for man.

Work was also done on augmentation of activity of chemotherapy by interferons in human malignant mesothelioma xenografts in nude mice by Sklarin and colleagues (1988).

I used intramuscular injections of interferon in the treatment of four cases of cancer using three mega units three times weekly. One case was mesothelioma and the other three abdominal carcinomas. The first (case M27) had a life expectancy of a few weeks when I began this treatment. He responded very well and was able to travel the following year. The X rays in Figure 6.2 show his condition before and after treatment.

The second X ray was performed after the fluid aspiration and a single infusion of bleomycin. Histological examination of these cells showed that they were both diastase negative and carcinogenic embryonic antigen (CEA) negative and cytokeratin positive, with the appearance of a malignant mesothelioma of the pleura (see Figure 6.3).

Because of my interest in the relationship between viruses and inorganic factors on the immune system and in malignant disease, the effects of interferons were known to me. Uncoated white asbestos fibers were the inorganic factors in this case. The patient had come intoclose contact with this material during his many years of employment in the shipyards.

FIGURE 6.2. X Rays Showing M27's Condition Before and After Treatment

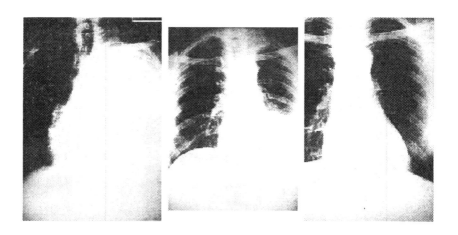

Before treatment   After aspiration   After interferon

FIGURE 6.3. Photomicrographs of Mesothelioma Stained with H & E at X75 and X187 Magnification

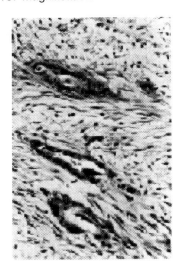 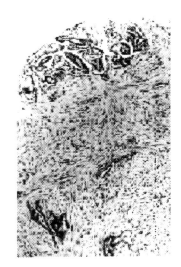

The other three cases of abdominal carcinoma are among those mentioned elsewhere. They occurred years after severe coxsackie infection and were of pancreatic origin. Two of these were unsuitable for surgery, and the other (case M28) had exploratory surgery that showed a diffuse retroperitoneal tumor spreading above the diaphragm into the mediastinum. This man's condition responded well to interferon therapy, but after his remission he died from an unrelated stroke. Both these cases improved so much during treatment that I recorded them on videotape.

Finally, we have to consider what the virion diseases such as transmissible spongiform encephalopathy (TSE) and prion protein (PrP) may teach us. Professor Lacey gave a good review of TSE at a lecture in Newcastle upon Tyne General Hospital. A normal form of this protein is found in normal CNS tissue and is coded by a gene in chromosome 2. PrP is highly conserved between species. Chromosome 2 encodes PrP messenger RNA. Initially, the protein is identical to natural protein but is modified to the infective form after production. It is found in the periplasm and has an affinity for joining liposomes or membranes and has been found in amyloid tissue. Affected bovine brain is expected to have 60 to 100 million infective units per gram. As shown previously, the actual infective dose can come from cumulative amounts in food. Peripheral nerves have been shown to contain PrP.

There is the possibility that Creutzfeldt-Jakob disease (CJD) and other motor neuron diseases originate in virus or prion infection. However, in CJD the evolution may be because of genetic predisposition or mutation, as I have described in coxsackie B virus disease. A high incidence of CJD occurs in Libyan Jews, which suggests genetic predisposition to exogenous infection. The crucial question that applies to all other agents is, "Is a high infectious dose required for the agent to enter a cell receptor?" If so, then small doses might be eliminated by the automimmune system and theoretically not pose such a risk. Exceptions would include people with impaired immunity, additive cofactors (either multiple viral infection or virus plus toxins with which the immune system is overloaded), or the possible persistence of virus or toxin that can be augmented by further exposure.

Excellent papers by Professors Roger Loria, David Ben-Nathan and Bracha Rager-Zisman were presented at the workshop of the Newcastle Research Group in April 1995 on host response to virus-mediated disease. They show in a very precise degree the host factors involved in resistance to viral infection.

Thus, it may be deduced that host reactions are of paramount importance for the prevention or recovery from illness no matter what the etiology and that these functions should be considered and utilized in both research and practice.

Chapter 7

Viral Effects in Pregnancy

Studies of the effects of viruses on pregnancy have been described in Chapter 4; however, the relationship of fetus to mother or mother to fetus is obviously delicate and complex. In Chapter 4, it was observed that a high proportion of members had equally high titers of the same virus as the patient, but without illness. Thus, the complexity of host reactions can be seen within families and is also relevant to this chapter on the outcomes in pregnancy. The overall perinatal mortality rate for England and Wales is 21 per 1,000 births in apparently "healthy" females; but this excludes deaths in the neonatal period as well as those later in the perinatal period. Many of these, as can be seen in other studies, are unexplained. If these figures, brief as they may be, are compared to the statistics later in this chapter, then a significant difference will be seen.

Butler and colleagues (1963) showed that nearly a fifth of such perinatal deaths were due to congenital malformations. Some idea of the incidence of deformities that might result from an epidemic is seen in the discussion by Cooper and colleagues (1969). They estimated that the rubella epidemic in 1964 resulted in 30,000 deformed babies. This did not take abortions into account. That different viruses may cause neonatal malformations is now well attested, but in this series the main offenders to be studied are enteroviruses, although syndromes due to other viruses are reported, including cytomegalovirus and rubella viruses. These viruses are transmitted through the placenta, and in series it will be obvious that many factors play a part in determining the damage to the fetus. Thus, as shown in Chapter 4, there is a real difference between infection and ensuing disease. In the pregnant patient there may be infection without apparent illness in the host, which may occur at the time of conception or even in the last trimester. Thus in the infected mother, during the period of embryogenesis varying effects on developing organs in the fetus may occur, while later in pregnancy fully developed organs would be affected. These effects will be discussed in the case presentations.

It has been obvious during this study that the degree of illness in the patient bears no real relationship to the severity of effects on the unborn child. This is also paralleled by the observation that the mere height of viral antibody titers in patients bears no real relationship to the severity of developing illness. From observations made during this study, it would appear that the significant factors that could affect the fetus are:

1. The actual time of the acute infection
2. The success or otherwise of the host immune-mediated response to the infection

From the study it appears that if the mother succumbed to some consequential illness, then it was more likely that the fetus would also be affected, bearing in mind that evidence of actual illness in the mother might be very slight. However, an ongoing postviral-mediated illness does not in itself appear to have any serious prognostications for pregnancy. Some patients who had a postpoliomyelitic syndrome (e.g., paralysis of one leg) gave birth to perfectly normal babies. In addition, there is a synergism between the fetus and the mother.

Many years ago, when dogs were used as models to investigate diabetes, the depancreatized, pregnant bitch was supported by the circulation of insulin derived from the fetus. For a similar reason, a number of patients in this study, where there was evidence of postviral-mediated syndromes (e.g., myalgic encephalomyelitis), the pregnant woman actually improved during pregnancy, but some lapsed afterward. This is the observation, but the interpretation may be somewhat obscure and might be related to neuroendocrine interdependent mechanisms. Thus it is true to say that a hazard to the fetus is not necessarily related to the degree of illness in the mother, but to the actual viral activity during the total period of pregnancy from conception to parturition.

The mother's immune system undoubtedly has a role to play in these circumstances. The numbers in this series are small, but none of those who were receiving intramuscular IgG at the time of conception and during pregnancy gave birth to a baby with any fetal abnormality. This observation is probably worthy of further trials. It is known that during parturition cytomegalovirus as well as the herpes groups and other viral infections may be transmitted to the fetus via the cervix, but in this study a transplacental passage appears to be the most likely route of infection, and hence protection gained from IgG, as delineated here, could be helpful.

For this study, 249 female patients of childbearing age—from seventeen to thirty-five years of age—were selected from data stored on the computer covering four decades. They all had had a viral illness sufficient to have viral screening tests performed, but the severity of the illness varied from mild to quite severe. This is evident in the case reports. They all had titers with at least a sixteenfold rise for enteroviruses and also positive IgM responses, but only sixty-six became pregnant during the infective period. Forty-five had normal babies (68.2 percent). As had been my practice for the last thirty years, I gave all the cases folate supplements at the commencement of pregnancy. All the mothers in the group with a normal outcome were also receiving IgG for their illness, although their serological titers still remained high. However, by the same token, twenty-one (31.8 percent), had an abnormal outcome, with 3.0 percent abortion, 9.1 percent stillbirths, and 16.7 percent with abnormalities. Another 3.0 percent also had continuing perinatal consequences, which resulted in death in subsequent months. None in this group had received IgG infusions. Compared to the neonatal morbidity rate for the general population, this statistical significance cannot be lightly dismissed (see Figure 7.1).

CASE REPORTS

Family 04

The case of Family 04 is also mentioned elsewhere. The mother was a housewife with a son and daughter and was the first member of the family to have a coxsackie-mediated illness in the form of viral meningitis. She made a good recovery. Her titers of coxsackie B group 4 were very high. After her recovery the titers fell, and she became pregnant. During the last trimester of pregnancy she had a relapse of her viral illness with another rise in antibody titers. However, the delivery was normal and the baby appeared normal at birth. Because of the viral illness I kept a close watch on the baby, and at about ten weeks he developed a systolic murmur. One of my pediatric colleagues

FIGURE 7.1. Analysis of Sixty-Six Actual Pregnancies from 249 Eligible Patients of Childbearing Age with High Coxsackie Titers

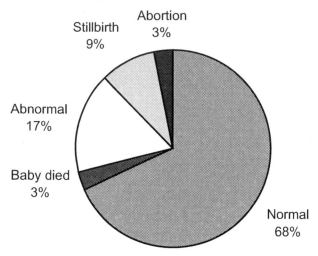

came to see him with me but thought that the murmur might be due to a congenital septum defect. As I had carefully assessed the baby since birth, and because of the recurring maternal illness, I felt that this was not so. Unfortunately, the baby went into congestive heart failure, and, though much was done to try to support him, he died in his first year. At postmortem examination, quite marked endocardial fibroelastosis was evident as the cause of the congestive heart failure and death. As discussed in Chapter 4, the whole family had high titers without illness. A year or two after this event, the woman's other son, who was by then about seventeen years of age, became ill. He had a recurrence of high titers of coxsackie B group 4, and this time had a severe viral myocarditis. He had to have a heart transplant and so far is well.

F18

Case F18 is similar in both history and outcome to the previous case. This young woman developed a severe facial palsy (Bell's palsy) and was also generally ill. As her coxsackie titers rose, similar to the case in Family 04, the details will be omitted. Her pregnancy and delivery were normal, and the baby's subsequent progress was identical to that of the previous case in that the baby developed a severe murmur and died before it was a year old. The photomicrograph of the interior of this baby's heart is identical to the first case of myocardial fibroelastosis as shown in Figure 4.3. The mother, however, went on to develop myalgic encephalomyelitis and was ill for some years, during which she developed recurring cysts of first one and then the other breast. I aspirated approximately 100 ml of clear fluid from one or two of these cysts and a smaller amount on other occasions. On laboratory examination nothing of note was found, and it is interesting that a woman currently under my care has had similar mammary cysts, as have others, but without any malignancy developing in any in this series.

F35

Case F35 is of considerable family interest, and occurred over thirty years ago. She was the mother of the following case (F36) and the sister of case M15 (discussed in Chapter 3). She became pregnant, and a Doppler scan at ten weeks gestation elicited a fetal heartbeat. Her expected date of delivery was then carefully calculated as September 19. She later developed a coxsackie viral illness and, while I was on holiday, she came to see my very competent assistant, as she had not felt movements for some days. On careful examination, he could not elicit a fetal heartbeat but suggested that she await my return. When I saw her the following week, I also found no fetal heartbeat on Doppler scan, and the uterine fundal height had regressed. One of my late expert obstetric colleagues (Dr. Frank Stabler) saw her with me. He felt that this was one of the very rare cases of "hibernation" and should be left to nature. She was regularly examined, and the fetal heartbeat became audible about six weeks after the initial cessation. She was ultimately delivered in November of that year and the baby was normal. This was a fascinating, happy outcome without morbid sequelae.

F36

F36 is the sister of the baby mentioned in case F35 and had a rather severe attack of Bornholm disease with similar high titers. In this case, as in others, I assisted a gynecological colleague with a laparoscopy, and we recovered about 300 cc of clear, straw-colored fluid, from which the virus was cultured. Shortly after this event she became pregnant but did not consult me until about the tenth week of gestation.

Hence I could not offer protection with IgG. The delivery, which I attended in the patient's home, was perfectly normal and resulted in an apparently healthy female with an Apgar score of 10. Once again, within days on this occasion, the baby developed a marked, diffuse cardiac murmur, and I referred her to a pediatric cardiological colleague. She was subjected to heart surgery because of multiple septal defects.

Family 01

The mother in Family 01 was, previous to marriage, a native of the Tyneside area. She came home from living abroad with her husband to see her parents. Her husband was not well (details appear as case M11 in Chapter 2). He had viral myocarditis, which went on to cardiomyopathy. This woman was also affected and had high titers of coxsackie B and had positive ELISA IgM and IgG when she became pregnant. They returned home, where sadly the husband died after their female baby was born. This baby had a large, flabby mouth and flabby limbs. These are apparent on the photographs as a baby and at age thirteen (see Figure 3.2).

The pediatricians in the hospital did all the possible tests, including genetic assessment, and nothing of note was found, but it was felt that she had an odd congenital amyotrophy. The hospital in their hometown kept me up-to-date with the child's progress and their findings. She survived to her early teens, but the amyotrophy was by then very marked. She could not walk and later was confined to bed and tube-fed. She died subsequently, with a pattern of disease seen in adults with progressive muscular dystrophy.

These five cases illustrate the ongoing effects on muscle tissue, both cardiac and skeletal, that have occurred in this series. The Coxsackieviruses and the ECHO strains have been recognized as causal agents of disease in both these tissues and have been recovered from them in biopsy specimens.

Family 05

The mother had a marked viral illness at approximately the eighth month of pregnancy. Viral screening was done, and ECHO virus was cultivated from the stools. The late Dr. P. Szekely, a cardiologist who had a special interest in heart disease during pregnancy, took an interest in her, as she also developed a perimyocarditis. Shortly after this initial event the fetal heart ceased, and she was delivered of a stillborn baby just about a week before her due date. Unfortunately, a postmortem examination was not carried out on the baby. To compound the issue, her husband then developed a coxsackie-mediated illness that later rendered him diabetic. As with others in this series, he had recurring attacks of pancreatitis, and some years later he developed carcinoma of the pancreas, from which he died.

F37

F37 had a rather severe viral illness while visiting her relatives at Christmas. She also was in her eighth month of pregnancy; in this case her third pregnancy. Her titers of coxsackie B group 4 demonstrated a sixteenfold rise, and she followed the pattern of the previous case with a stillborn female baby, without overt signs of abnormality. As with the previous case, due to emotional issues postmortem examination was not performed. She did not recover well from this episode and had a mild psychotic type of illness. It was felt that this could well have been a sequel to the viral illness rather than being related to the unfortunate outcome of the pregnancy.

F15

F15 was in the twenty-fourth week of her third pregnancy and came to my surgery feeling vaguely unwell. Blood pressure and general examination revealed little except that her urine contained urobilinogen. An examination was repeated the following day with the same results, and blood was taken for viral screening. It showed the rise in titers stated as diagnostic for coxsackie B group 4. She was hospitalized, but sadly, within a week the fetal heart arrested and she had a stillbirth; more sadly still, she herself went on to hepatorenal failure and had to be transferred to the intensive care unit where, after a stormy illness, she died.

These three cases represent some of the cases that resulted in stillbirth from enteroviral infection, and the other possible disastrous consequences that may ensue either in the actual host or some other member of the immediate family.

F38

Patient F38 gave birth to twin boys during the 1960s. She had an attack of Bornholm disease prior to conception. The births were uneventful, and the twins appeared normal. I was called to see one of the boys when he was eight months of age, as he had had an epileptic fit. He was seen by a pediatric colleague. At that time his mother was given barbiturate medication for him and further investigation was arranged. However, she was unhappy about this and did not give him the medicine. He had another fit about a week later and died. A postmortem was carried out, showing that he had an arrest of renal development at the mesonephros stage. We believed that the renal tissue had been sufficient to support his body mass up to a certain weight, but then failed, and due to this failure all the other consequences ensued. The other twin is still well thirty years later, and his intravenous pyelogram (IVP), which was done as a precaution, was normal. The question here is why only one should succumb, and so far we have failed to find any answer. There were two separate placentas, but whether this had any relevance was, and still is, sub judice. This case probably represents one of the rare cases of an arrest of organ development.

The following case reports illustrate some of the central nervous system defects where infection occurred during pregnancy. The first case was due to infection in the last trimester.

F39

F39 is the mother of case M20 (see Chapter 3). She became pregnant and was fit and well until the eighth month, when she had a very severe attack of Bornholm disease with severe abdominal cramping. A possible diagnosis of abruptio placentae was suggested. The pain remitted after a day or so and, as so often happens, recurred a week later with additional force. Her serological titers followed the pattern alluded to earlier, and a stool viral culture was positive. Her labor was normal. This was in 1977, and based on my experience, I undertook careful assessment of cardiac and neurological systems. At about fourteen weeks I considered that the baby's developing reflexes were not symmetrical. My pediatric colleague cooperated and a CAT scan was performed. (Actually, I think he was the first baby to have a CAT scan at the hospital.) The results demonstrated on the CAT scan have been verified in recent years by an MRI scan. This shows a considerable erosion of brain tissue. However, apart from some weakness in the upper limbs, he had good attendance at school and was treated more or less as a normal boy. It is interesting that he recently passed his car driving test. Obviously, all that he learned from birth onward has been "written" on the surviving, intact brain tissue and thus is available, whereas had this trauma occurred later in life there would have been more disastrous results. This case was presented in the *Lancet* in 1968.

The following cases illustrate the possible effects of first-trimester viral infection.

Family 02

The mother in Family 02, like some of the other cases, had an illness of similar viral etiology and subsequent titer profiles confirmed this. She became pregnant while she had high titers and had an apparently normal pregnancy and delivery. No abnormality was noted at the time of delivery, which in this case was in the hospital. At postnatal examination all was apparently normal, but shortly afterward she felt that the baby was not responding to light and movement as he should. At an extensive interview, which I recorded on videotape, her observations were confirmed, and an MRI scan was arranged through the Newcastle Research Group. The results are shown in Chapter 4 (Figure 4.1) and demonstrate an agenesis of the septum pellucidum. He is very fond of music and though scarcely of school age, he sings and claps his hands to musical rhythm, which has been captured on videotape.

Family 03

The mother in Family 03 was a primipara and also had coxsackie B viral infection but was not significantly ill. This occurred late in 1982. Her titers of coxsackie B group 4 were above 1/512, and she had a positive ELISA IgM, and so fit into the same pattern as the others. The pregnancy was uneventful, and she delivered an apparently healthy female baby in the hospital on July 1983. Once again, the postnatal examination was normal and baby seemed fine. Despite careful examination of cardiovascular and central nervous systems all seemed normal for several months, when the mother felt that her child's responses and development were not satisfactory. After considerable observation and many examinations, I felt that a lack of myelin development was most likely, as there was no localized loss of function. Later an MRI was arranged, as shown in Chapter 4 (Figure 4.2). Sadly, by age ten, she has not developed in either mental or physical behavior. This overall abnormality can only be attributed to a general lack of development of myelin, with the resulting loss of communication within the brain tissue.

F40

The son of F40 is now in his twenties, and the case is mentioned to show that "white matter" agenesis, as seen in the previous two cases, is not all that rare. The mother had a similar mild viral illness just prior to conception and though not really ill, her titers of Coxsackievirus were high. The family lived on a housing estate where there was an "end-arterial" water supply, and in that decade quite a number of residents were ill due to the same strain of virus. She was a primigravida and the prenatal examinations were all normal. The hospital delivery was somewhat slow. Subsequent progress at first seemed normal but, as with the previous cases, a lack of coordination became increasingly evident. Later a CAT scan demonstrated agenesis of the corpus callosum. Though now in his twenties, and of considerable physique, he has widespread motor disorders and also suffers from epilepsy. He has been the subject of extensive investigation and much work has gone into helping him. It is interesting that he is addicted to music. He plays tapes for hours on end and sings lustily into a microphone, mimicking the performers whom he adulates. It is fascinating that he knows precisely the items on each tape and can find them more quickly than his parents. Apart from epilepsy and a lack of academic learning, motor disorders chiefly due to incoordination seem to predominate in his case.

F41

Twenty years ago, during an epidemic of rubella, F41 was in the last trimester of her first pregnancy. She was thirty-two years of age, very healthy and looking forward to having the baby. Unhappily she developed rubella. It was obvious that an abortion would not solve any problem, but I had to warn her of the possibility of a hearing deficit occurring. Once again the delivery and subsequent progress were normal. No doubt due to my warning, she watched for and noted a lack of directional eye movements to sounds fairly early in infancy. This was confirmed over the years, but the boy also became a happy, healthy young man and has done well academically. Varying means are being investigated for helping with his hearing deficit. Oddly enough, this is the only case in forty years that I can directly attribute to the rubella virus.

F42

F42 had a mild enteroviral infection, after which she became pregnant. All seemed well and the delivery was normal. At birth, however, the baby was found to have bilateral coloboma. She is now quite a fine schoolgirl and does not appear to have any other defect.

This case is reported as there was evidence of enteroviral infection at the time of conception. Other cases of cleft palate and harelip have occurred and also one case of abortion in which the facial cleft did not fuse, which is still preserved in a liquid medium. However, in most of these cases no illness was evident, and hence no titers were performed. During the four decades since 1955, more than 5,000 pregnancies have been carefully monitored, and I was responsible for most deliveries. During this time the usual abnormalities have been seen. Many of these were due to a lack of first-trimester development, including such syndromes as spina bifida, hydrocephalus due to lack of development of the basal cranial foramen, as well as other anomalies already mentioned.

Around this time, more than thirty years ago during an epidemic of Coxsackievirus-mediated illness, I was interested in the viral profile. Also, a fairly full blood screen was performed that included the usual serological cell types. Liver function tests together with assays of albumin and folate status were also performed. It was a little surprising that a fall in folate level was noted after some but not all of these viral illnesses. Moreover, there did appear to be some correlation between the severity of the illness and the degree of fall of the folate level. However, it was noted that the actual height of the serological antibody titer did not signify the severity of the ensuing illness. Knowing these facts, it was assumed that there was some significance.

From that time onward, I gave folic acid supplements to all the pregnant patients who consulted me. Most of them came to see me as soon as they missed one period. None of those who had this supplement early had a baby with spina bifida. Thus a question arises about the cause of the low folate level in the first place. In surveying the abnormalities reported where a rather severe viral infection resulted in maternal illness, most of the mothers had been given folate supplements. The exceptions were cases F37 and the mother in Family 01 (who had her baby in the United States). Moreover, there does appear to be a possible difference in ensuing pathology in abnormalities occurring during the first and later trimesters. Thus it may be possible that in the first trimester a viral infection that lowers folic acid could exert its effect indirectly by depriving the host of essential nutrients needed for cell development in the fetus; whereas after this development has occurred, a virus would cause pathology to mature organs.

However, this is not certain from the pregnancies discussed, though the patients had a significant illness. Most were given folate supplements, yet as shown, there were fetal abnormalities, but no spina bifida babies. Moreover, as stated earlier, none who had been "protected" by the use of IgG had an abnormal baby. Whether this had a direct sequential effect remains a question. Does the IgG, through immunological strategies, nullify the virus, and does this in turn halt any further pathological response, of which the folate profile might be just one indicator?

It is almost certain that there are multiple causes of fetal abnormality. Genetic defects are sought (e.g., Down's syndrome) and there is evidence that with increasing maternal age Down's syndrome is more likely to occur. However, the reason for the gene abnormality and whether increased age of the mother makes the gene more susceptible are still unknown. In this series, as far as I know, the question of inherited genetic reasons for fetal abnormalities did not arise, yet it is obvious that the actual pathological modus operandi is still not certain and may involve genetic "trauma," either by viruses or other substances (e.g., toxins), or possibly by the additive effects of both. Thus the reference to Down's syndrome is appropriate, as it is possible that the normal genetic sequences were changed, perhaps due to viral activity.

More could be said about the effects of viruses on organ development and development of other cell lines. Adelstein and Donovan (1972) and also Fedrick and Alberman (1982) showed a link between viral infection and childhood leukemia. A very full chapter in Szentivanyi and Friedman's (1986) book on viruses deals with the interactions between viruses and the immune system. As an illustration of this complexity, one case that does not appear elsewhere may be mentioned briefly. This patient had a mild to moderate illness with very high titers (<1,000) of coxsackie B virus both groups 2 and 4 and also a positive ELISA IgM test. She became pregnant, which was confirmed by a CAT scan, but she aborted an empty sac at about the eighth week of gestation. Months later, when she still had high titers, she again became pregnant, but this time a normal delivery resulted in an apparently normal baby. Sadly this child developed leukemia. This patient was not among those protected at the time of pregnancy by IgG.

Much more remains to be elucidated, as it is far from easy to define cause and effect. The observation of helper-suppressor cell ratios, in which the suppressor cells may predominate as a consequence of viral activity, is a fair example, for it is assumed that this is an abnormal and unhelpful host response. However, the converse may be true; if high levels of T cells (NK cells) were active, then large numbers of infected host cells would be destroyed, which could be catastrophic to the host. Thus it is possible that this helper-suppressor cell ratio reversal is possibly a host protective mechanism. Blumberg and colleagues (1967) reported on the Australian antigen (AuA) in both Down's syndrome and leukemia. They postulated that this AuA was located on a virus also. As the matter of genomic drift from viruses has been discussed, it would appear feasible to consider the possibility that such "drift" from an infecting virus would result in genetic acquisition of AuA, which would result in the adverse effects already shown.

It is obvious that many viruses can adversely affect fetal development. This study focuses mainly on the part played by enteroviruses. Maybe their role has not been as well recognized as it ought to be and more work should be done. Other factors have been studied, including not only the effects of viral infection but also those of toxins. The effects of thalidomide on the host are a good example. They do not appear to be as simple as they have been assumed to be. Without going into details, it is probable that the effects were also autoimmune mediated. In rats given thalidomide, it has been shown that the abortion rate falls by the amount of rise in fetal abnormality. Thus thalidomide appeared to prevent abortion but may not have been the actual cause of the fetal abnormality. Thalidomide is used currently for its beneficial, suppressive autoimmune effect in conditions such as nodular leprosy. Thus, autoimmune inhibition may have widely differing effects. As usual, we end up with more questions than answers.

Chapter 8
Neoplastic Sequelae

In this forty-year study, it appears to be significant that organs involved in neoplastic change were confined almost exclusively to the central nervous system and retroperitoneal regions. Some of these are surveyed anecdotally in Chapters 3 and 5.

In the CNS group, cerebral tumors predominated among males. There were ten in males compared to four in females, but in the latter there was one malignancy involving the lumbar plexus. Retroperitoneal malignancies were all confined to the pancreas and occurred in eight males (11.0 percent of male deaths), and six females (14.6 percent of female deaths).

Historically, neoplastic changes were not evident for approximately two to four years following the initial, severe viral illness. In the retroperitoneal group, all of the patients initially developed pancreatitis without diabetes. In 30 percent, this tended to recur months or years later, before neoplastic changes became evident. Weight loss and dull, persistent abdominal and lumbar pain were alerting factors. The CNS neoplastic sequelae were clinically much more subtle, and symptoms varied; in some a constant headache developed, while in others, mental deterioration was more evident. This deterioration manifested in some by cognitive changes and in others by somatic effects, of which dysergia was a relatively common finding. In these cases, weight loss was not a feature, but distress and the cognitive and somatic symptoms were the usual signals of possible malignancy.

Neoplastic changes do not reflect the initiating organic illness, and the sequelae in some cases were as follows: Bornholm disease with subsequent myocarditis, which remitted, and later still, encephalomyelitis with a cerebral tumor developing some years later. Other cases began in a similar fashion, and some developed cardiac symptoms that also remitted, but they did not fully recover and developed evidence of abdominal pathology. In some cases, irritable bowel syndrome occurred and, as in case F32 (Chapter 5), a peculiar and perplexing bowel disorder resulted. It was in this group that retroperitoneal carcinoma developed. The initiating illness, which in some cases involved the heart, had remitted, and the actual cause of death was the subsequent carcinoma. Doubtless it would be easy for the physician not to relate the terminal malignancy to the preceding illnesses.

From past experience, carcinogenic agents may be both organic and inorganic elements. Examples of organic elements include leukemia viruses, while the benzpyrine inhaled by cigarette smokers should be well known for its carcinogenic effects. Similarly, the mesotheliomas developing in those who have worked with asbestos demonstrate sinister, very late, sequelae from contact with inorganic elements. The effects of other inorganic elements, such as organophosphates, etc., will no doubt warrant inclusion in this category. This study has concentrated mainly on the effects of viruses, but over the years carcinoma of the lung and also the kidneys in cigarette smokers has occurred with the usual prevalence. Several cases of malignancy due to asbestos have been seen, and one is reported in detail in Chapter 6 as case M27.

CASE REPORTS

As this study is confined to the effects of viruses, the case reports analyzed here relate only to those of viral origin. The distribution of cases included in Group 5 in this study is shown in Table 8.1.

Analyzing these, it is apparent that in females the total CNS mortality was significantly greater than in males, while the cardiovascular mortality was correspondingly higher among males. However, in this study of malignancy, it is significant that there is no statistical

TABLE 8.1. Number of Cases in Group 5 and Cause of Death

	Female	%	Male	%
Total deaths	37		73	
CNS	11	30	8	11
CVS	16	43	47	64
Cancer	**10**	**27**	**18**	**25**
CNS malignancy	4	40	10	56
Retroperitoneal	6	60	8	44

difference in the total percentage of cases, though the CNS cases tend to predominate among males and the retroperitoneal cases among females. This is perhaps an unexpected result, but the significance should be considered with caution since the total numbers are not great.

The detailed case reports relating to these statistics are discussed in other chapters. Some cases not discussed elsewhere are of special interest here.

F43

F43 was twenty years old and had suffered from a viral illness, confirmed by the usual evidence of titers IgM, IgG, etc. About one to two years after the initial illness, she had what was considered to be "food aversion" and later was diagnosed as anorexia nervosa. I was called to see her one night and found her in bed with disequilibrium and complaining of constant headache. Her peripheral reflexes were unremarkable and she had obviously lost a little weight, but otherwise no distinct pathological pattern was apparent. Funduscopy did reveal bilateral, marginally congested optic disks. This was worrisome, and immediate in-depth investigations with MRI imaging were instituted. The outcome was evidence of a spreading glioma, which unfortunately was too diffuse to be removed by operation, and she died.

F44

F44, a thirty-six-year-old, was a very similar to F43, with similar serological evidence of persisting viral infection. The infection was confirmed by a persistently high VP1 test. She also had anorexia and nausea together with marked disequilibrium and balance problems. She was videotaped, and the tape is retained. A biopsy of her brain was attempted but did not yield a positive result, and her retinal fundi did not show evidence of pressure change as in case F43. However, she died, and at autopsy a fine, spreading astrocytoma was found.

M29

M29, a man in his early forties, had a typical Bornholm disease during the 1960s, from which he apparently recovered. Approximately two years later he began to complain of nausea and lack of appetite with food aversion and sporadic vomiting. One of my surgical colleagues investigated and performed a gastroenterostomy. Though there was no evidence of gastric pathology for a few weeks, he did not vomit but still had the food aversion. A vague suggestion that this might be anorexia nervosa did not appeal to me. Neither headache nor disequilibrium were marked features in this case, but he did show evidence of impaired mental function and discomfort. His deterioration was rapid and he died. At autopsy, a fairly widespread glioma was seen but no abdominal malignancy.

M30

M30, a fifty-year-old man, had an acute attack of viral meningitis in the 1970s. The usual investigations showed serological evidence for coxsackie B group 4. He recovered and appeared well for approximately two years. In contrast to the previous case, he did not develop anorexia but did have marked disequilibrium, dysergia, mild nystagmus, and evidence of impaired motor function, chiefly of the upper limbs. This progressed over months, but unfortunately we did not have access to MRI scans and the CAT scan was not well defined. He became totally bedridden, and, though it was difficult to visualize his fundi, the optic disks showed some signs of blurring. After thorough investigations had been completed, it was felt that an operation would not be helpful, and he also died. The subsequent autopsy showed a rather diffuse glioma affecting chiefly the midbrain.

F45

One case in the 1950s was remarkable in that the patient first lost her sense of smell. This occurred about a year after a meningeal illness of coxsackie origin. This was confirmed by stool culture of the virus as well as serological evidence of its persistence over months. Later there was evidence of cranial nerve pathology spreading from the first anterior cranial nerve nuclei, that is, the olfactory nerve, to the twelfth cranial nerve in the posterior nuclei. There was a sequential involvement of the trochlea, then the abducens, and later still the glossopharyngeal nerve nuclei, with consequential focusing and swallowing difficulties. This woman was only in her forties when she died, and the autopsy revealed a spreading cerebral tumor.

Over the years, these cases have suggested that symptoms of disequilibrium, dysergia, imbalance, and anorexia, should be viewed as possible evidence of serious intracranial pathology. Other cases with identical symptoms and of the same viral origin have occurred. Some of these died due to severe, cellular brain pathology, but no malignancy was evident.

In two other cases, it was possible to operate on the tumor and, so far, the patients are surviving free of persisting symptoms. One of these cases was a member of a three-generation family (Family 06; see Chapter 4). Later, she herself had a daughter, and all four generations died of coxsackie infection. This patient developed acromegaly but, unfortunately, this preceded the surgical removal of the tumor. Moreover, there is only familial evidence that this tumor may have had a viral origin.

These cases, while limited in number, are sufficiently indicative of varying pathology to warrant further research into the association of etiological mechanisms, particularly where malignancy occurs.

Chapter 9

Treatment Considerations

Sublata causa tollitur effectus—remove the cause and the effect will cease—may be true in some illnesses but not in all. It depends upon the degree of tissue damage as well as the varying regeneration ability of different tissues. Thus a holistic approach is needed to halt the pathogenic process, which could be viral, bacterial, inorganic, or autoimmune, and then to aid the tissue repair if possible. Dealing with the cellular mechanisms in viral infections, we can consider then the substrate that is infected and also the varying host mechanisms invoked to deal with the infection and repair.

CELLULAR CONSIDERATIONS

The cell map shown in Figure 9.1 demonstrates the complexity of the possible local response. Essential fatty acids are involved and have been shown to fail after viral infection (Williams et al.) Their functions are threefold:

1. They are structural components of the cell membrane.
2. They are precursors of prostaglandins and interleukins.
3. They play a part in the transport and oxidation of cholesterol and lipids.

A simple overview of their synthesis and function follows.

Membrane Mediators

1. They act on receptors and are necessary for enzyme function.
2. They act as messengers during a chainlike conversion as follows:

   a. From linoleic acid. Genetic dysfunction can possibly occur here. This desaturates to:

FIGURE 9.1. Cell Map

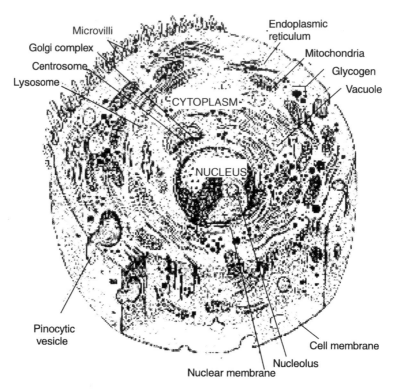

Microvilli
Golgi complex
Centrosome
Lysosome
Endoplasmic reticulum
Mitochondria
Glycogen
Vacuole
CYTOPLASM
NUCLEUS
Pinocytic vesicle
Cell membrane
Nucleolus
Nuclear membrane

b. Gammalinoleic acid, which is further desaturated to:
c. Dihormogammalinoleic acid, which in turn is converted to eicosanoids, which is the first chain reaction in interferon activity, which results in:
d. Prostaglandins, which are the essential outcome of the cyclo-oxygenase system and are intimately linked with interferon function.

Interferon Activity

1. Interferon activity may be inhibited if linoleic acid is not converted to gammalinoleic acid. Generally this is due to a genetic cause.
2. If cyclooxygenase is lacking, interferon/prostaglandin synthesis is inhibited.

Interferon itself is inactive in cell lines lacking the enzyme cyclo-oxygenase (Chandrobose et al., 1981). EFAs are substrates for this enzyme. EFAs are also essential substrates in muscle oxidative phosphorylation and neuronal metabolism. Replicating viruses can directly use host lipids and so deprive host cells of EFAs. As EFAs are synthesized in the liver microsomes, any hepatic insult would affect EFAs throughout the body. Whatever the varying mechanisms may be, it does appear rational to augment the host's own synthesis of EFAs. Studies have shown a subjective response to EFAs of about 80 percent compared to 18 percent in a placebo group.

As Paul Levine also noted, and was mentioned at the Cambridge symposium (Hyde, Biddle, and McNamara, 1991), other trigger factors can play a role in determining the pathological effect of a virus. They may be related to the state of the autoimmune system at the time. It should be borne in mind that the autoimmune functions of the body are determined by B and T cells, but they do not operate in the brain above the basal ganglia area. The astrocytes generally are the caretakers of immune function at higher brain levels.

Moreover, the blood-brain barrier (BBB) is known to function in relation to lipids, and by and large, only lipid-soluble substances can pass the BBB. The thalamic and hypothalamic areas are not protected by the BBB. It is perhaps rather ironic that viruses, being lipid soluble, can pass the BBB and cause havoc in the higher cortex as well as invading the hypothalamic area. MRI imaging that we and others (Royce Biddle MD, Stockton, California) have done demonstrates, in a number of ME cases, the so-called UBOs which occur in areas of arterial supply to the brain and are not scattered like the plaques we see in multiple sclerosis. Hyde, Biddle, and McNamara (1991) suggested that these were in the Virchow-Robin (VR) spaces that surround the blood vessels. In a case of mine that was autopsied, virus was found in these spaces. Also, WBCs were found in the CSF surrounding the cerebral arteries, that is, in the VR spaces.

The hypothalamic area does indeed depend on the general body immune mediation by T and B cells, whereas the higher centers by and large depend on the astrocytes, in some infective states, there could be an invasion of the BBB by peripheral WBCs.

The lipid substrates also contain a mechanism for the passage of the BBB. Choline dihydrogen citrate has for decades been known to affect the deposition of fat in the liver, or, viewed in another way, to actively help metabolize the hepatic lipids. It mobilizes lipids in any area, including the intima of blood vessels and also any lipid coating on bacteria or virus or toxin. Ascorbic acid used in conjunction with this sulfonates and renders the lipids water soluble and facilitates renal excretion. Thus this mixture can act synergistically with the EFAs and obviously passes the BBB. It is also a precursor of acetylcholine, one of the neurotransmitter enzymes. There is a role for its effect during the infective stage and a continuing role in the repair stages.

AUTOIMMUNE MECHANISMS

It is relevant that there are not only circulating antibodies but also local organ-related antibodies. This might well be a factor in reducing specificity as well as the number of organs affected. This applies mainly to areas other than those above the BBB. In 25 percent of ME or postviral mediated and ongoing chronic syndromes, organ-specific antibodies occur (e.g., antithyroid antibodies). These should be viewed as part of the host response, which may relate to a protective function or be idiotypic and therefore detrimental. This local organ antibody activity was seen in a study of a series of infertile women. This activity was recorded on video and demonstrates intense activity by cervical mucosal cells, which within a minute of exposure attacked, deformed, and killed sperm. From the same samples, sperm incubated overnight in serum from the women survived normally, thus showing that the antibodies were not in general circulation.

Another consideration is that the search for a definitive virus may be confusing, for it is well known that infection with one defined virus may have a resurgent effect on a latent virus, which may in turn have a more pathological effect.

It can also be shown that things which appear to occur in parallel cannot always be viewed simply as cause and effect, but may be synergistic. A good example is seen in a review in the *British Medical Journal* (Vol. 307, October 1993, p. 832), which looked at the association between diabetes and lipoproteins in relation to coronary heart disease. The authors admitted that both of these had some relationship to coronary heart disease and in that sense were synergistic but failed to find an actual causal relationship between the two factors. Loria's (1986a) work, on the other hand, goes into more detail and emphasizes the synergism between these factors.

> Coxsackie B virus and lipids are common synergistic determinants in diabetes and atherosclerosis. Their independent and synergistic interactions suppress host immunity. It is estimated that of all those who have a significant illness due to coxsackie B virus, 5 percent will have some post viral mediated pathology, be it cardiomyopathy or some other syndrome. The coxsackie B virus has no envelope and no lipid in its capsule. It can cause fat necrosis in the host and in culture medium intracellular cholesterol crystals are found. In virus infected cells there is an increase in the incorporation of choline in phospholipids and this may well be part of a protective attempt to flush the lipids in which virus is found.

Any genetic lack, Loria considered, should be viewed as a host inability to synergistically produce antibodies that are either serological or organ specific. He showed that atherosclerosis is higher in diabetics and is related to mortality in 75 percent, but he proceeded to show in mice that hypercholesterolemia itself was not necessarily associated with atheromatous changes.

However, if these mice with high lipids were infected with coxsackie B virus, a 97 percent mortality occurred in two weeks due to cardiomyopathy. The virus was found in the aortic tissue. Histological examination months later showed endothelial cell swelling and disruption of medial cells with lipidlike vacuolation. Neither the infected normocholesterolemic mice nor the uninfected hypercholesterolemic mice developed atherosclerotic lesions. However, hypercholesterolemia was shown to have a marked immunosuppressive effect, which extended to tumerigenesis, via the virus-induced "sick cell syndrome."

Jay Goldstein looked at IL-2 and T-8 receptor levels as well as NK cell function because the serological levels of the latter are often lowered. If IL-2 was raised, he thought the patient would respond to IgG treatment. Professor Roger Loria (1992) has done some excellent work on the protective effect of androstenediol (AED) in BALB mice that were infected with Coxsackievirus. Since 1996, Professor Loria has done additional work that shows the further changes in the steroid chain which result in AED being superceded by the trials (i.e., androestenetriol, AET), which have a much more potent protective effect against viral invasion. It is not yet being used in humans but holds out definite hope for a further host approach.

Overall, it would seem logical to use host mechanisms, and this needs much more in-depth study. However, currently IgG infusion can be used as an immunological approach. This was used by Lord Horder in 1929 with dramatic effect in relation to viral encephalitis. There is a steady accumulation of evidence for its role in more diverse syndromes where infective and autoimmune mechanisms play a therapeutic role.

Meanwhile, I use IgG by intramuscular infusion where there is evidence of virus-induced, abnormal immunological response. Analysis of responses to a questionnaire completed by many patients receiving this treatment shows an 80 percent definite subjective improvement. Of the other 20 percent, half felt unchanged and half just "did not know." However, the objective signs of improvement were demonstrable in several cases of quite marked myocarditis, where the ECG normalized after this treatment.

In one case when the IgG treatment was discontinued too early, the ECG again became abnormal, as it was prior to treatment. This raises a question about the criteria for commencing and then discontinuing infusions of IgG. Serological evidence for persistent virus-mediated illness is seen in positive ELISA IgG and VP1 tests. In these circumstances, treatment with IgG should begin. It continues while the tests remain positive but, in my opinion, a subsequent negative VP1 test merely demonstrates a lack of persisting viral infection but does not rule out a latent, nonproliferating viral infection. When the tests become negative and remain so on three successive occasions at monthly intervals, then IgG treatment may be discontinued. In some cases, the cessation of IgG infusions was followed by the return of a positive VP1 test. This was also shown by Professor J. Mowbray (Jenkins and Mowbray, 1991).

Interrelating genetic malfunction with viral infection may have a hidden cause. Many years ago, a student of mine was given an ME case to study. She wrote a short thesis, having looked at relevant research including one paper that suggested a faulty gene on chromosome 21 as one of the determining factors in succumbing to the illness (Khesin et al., 1978). This work suggested that the acquisition of resistance to coxsackie B viruses by cells accompanied by characteristic changes in cell metabolism, coupled with a decrease in the number of small chromosomes of the G group, i.e., pairs 21 and 22, was most constantly observed. In about 20 percent of the resistant cells in whose chromosome sets G21 was still present, there was reason to suppose that these chromosomes, or at least their loci connected with coding of the cell receptors to coxsackie B virus, were in a state of deep repression. In their view, preservation of physiological interchromosomal interactions played an important role in the objective study of the nature and mechanisms of specific resistance of cells to viruses. This is supported by work by Ferdinando Dianzani et al. (1988) in which they showed that human IFNα and IFNβ share a common receptor, which was coded for by chromosome 21.

Various questions could be asked about nucleic, mitochondrial, and diverse genetic functions. It is possible that, in varying degrees, each one of these areas may be affected. It has been shown that melatonin exerts a protective effect against DNA damage by free radicals and enhances antibody response to infection (Reiter, 1994). Thus we are probably dealing with diverse intracellular pathological mechanisms. How can this be related to treatment? At the moment, the immunomodulatory effects of IgG appear to be the most effective, comprehensive treatment available.

The protective effects of substances as diverse as melatonin and dihydroandroanediol (DHEA) may point the way to other strategies. As more research is undertaken into this complex subject, no doubt more refined treatments will be developed.

ESSENTIAL FATTY ACIDS IN CIRCULATION AND CELL MEMBRANE

As shown earlier, during viral infection choline is absorbed into lipids where virus particles are found. This should be viewed as a host response. Many years ago, this substance was used in the treatment of diphtheria and was shown to prevent fatty deposition in the liver and also had a protective effect on the development of diptheritic myocarditis. The sinusoids and Kupffer cells in the liver are probably loci of viral infection, and thus the mobilization of lipids would result in sequestration of these loci.

As cells depend largely on membrane activity for healthy function, it would appear logical to utilize therapy that would preserve or restore this integrity, and the essential fatty acids have been shown to play an important role here.

Choline also plays an intercessory role as a precursor of acetylcholine in the CNS and also greatly ameliorates the effects of atherosclerosis with all its attendant risks, which play an important part in the development of varying pathological states.

I conducted a study over a five-year period involving 426 patients with an average age of forty-eight years, who all displayed a high level of serum cholesterol. By the calibration then applied, a "safe level" was considered to be 225, and most of the patients had initial levels exceeding 300.

- Thirty-six patients were treated with clofibrate alone (twenty-eight males and eight females). In this group, four patients suffered strokes, and this treatment was discontinued in thirty-two cases.
- Seventy-six patients who were initially treated with clofibrate were subsequently supplemented with choline.
- Three hundred fourteen patients were treated with choline alone.

As can be seen from Figure 9.2, the administration of choline alone often resulted in an initial rise of serum cholesterol. Presumably, this was due to the mobilization of lipid deposits. This was invariably followed by a steady decline in serum cholesterol to safe levels when the mobilization was complete. This was accompanied in some by the disappearance of a soft arcus and, in two females, by the clearing of carotid bruits. Statistically, considering the varying pathology in all these cases, twenty major events were forecast but only the four mentioned occurred.

These cases are cited to show the effects of a choline dihydrogen citrate/ascorbic acid mixture on cholesterol. The cases themselves had varied pathology including viral myocarditis, coronary and other artery diseases, as well as virus-mediated CNS syndromes and diabetes.

FIGURE 9.2. Effects of Clofibrate and Choline on Serum Cholesterol

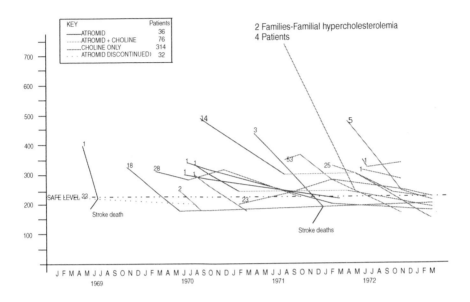

VACCINATION

Eventually, as with poliomyelitis, the question of vaccination must arise. It has been considered for decades, but as the number of enteroviruses capable of inducing these syndromes is over seventy, in contrast to the three of polio, it is not easy. However, with the common factors of VP1 etc. now emerging, together with certain other common strand material, this may be a possibility for the near future and could well prevent a great deal of illness, from juvenile diabetes to cardiomyopathy.

Coxsackie B group 3 has been shown to be cardiotoxic by Reihnard Kandolf (1988) and, very recently, was the subject of a paper by Professor Len Archard at a Newcastle Research Group conference.

The coxsackie B virus group has no envelope and do not have lipid in their capsid, but are known for their lipotoxic qualities and their ability to cause fat necrosis. However, in tissue culture, they cause the formation of intracellular cholesterol crystals. Virus infection results in an increased cellular incorporation of choline in phospholipids, which is associated with virus-induced infection in membrane structures in the centrosphere region of infected cells.

R. B. Herberman (1986) shows that viruses and tumors have an effect on the immune system and vice versa. In an updated version of immune surveillance, he suggests:

> Tumor cells and microbial agents, or cells infected by such agents, have surface markers recognized by one or more effectors. These target cells will be susceptible to lysis or growth inhibition by this effector mechanism. It can induce a febrile response which inhibits replication. It enhances phagocytosis, activates immune killer cell (NK) elements. It sensitizes infected cells to antibody dependent immunolysis. It induces other lymphokines to act in synergy to lyse infected cells.

Once again, it is not simple. Eradication of virus from cells by interferons is good. However, where virus has gained access and is in the cell, then interferon augmentation of immunolysis could be harmful. For example, in the brain, where a "slow viral" syndrome is operative and perhaps most cells contain virus, the lysing of all these cells could be disastrous. The patient would be left with no infected cells, but also with no brain! This would not apply, however, to the lysis of cancer by interferons, as only cancer cells would be affected.

Interferons are part of the immune system, which is influenced by the thymus. Thymic humoral factor takes part in T cell differentiation in lymphoid cells, in the thymus itself, in bone marrow, and in lymph glands. It regulates thymocytes and T cells in the absence of antibody stimulation. It thus helps maintain the balance of T helper, T suppressor and T cytotoxic (NK) cells. Thus far we can say the biological activity of THF will:

1. Promote hemopoiesis
2. Increase helper effect of T cells in the production of antibodies and increase reactivity to mitogens
3. Augment T cell NK effects against syngenic tumors
4. Increase secretion of interleukin 2 by T cells
5. Restore balance of T helper/suppressor cells when it is impaired

The question is how to be specific in stimulating or suppressing activity of cell types. The lymphocytokines are highly potent and active at minute levels. Cultured cell lines are now possible and the production of lymphocytokines quantitatively improved. Lymphoblastoid interferon (Welferon) is a lymphocytokine. There are twenty known varieties of interferons coded for by fifteen different genes, as well as beta and gamma interferons. We need to know the action of each mediator and where it is appropriate. The National Cancer Institute has shown that interleukin 2 in common with interferon stimulates NK activity. Also, alpha interferon, as well as having antiviral activity, has antitumor activity across a variety of tumors.

It seems that viruses or virions in cells can induce interferon activity; but depending on whether the infection is early, late, or secondary, then alpha, beta, or gamma interferon is produced. The role of the interferon activity at varying levels needs to be understood as we are dealing with potent mechanisms. Interferons must be considered at many stages of infection, including the primary portal, the secondary foci, the circulating system, and the terminal target tissues. They have the following actions:

1. Reduce virus attachment or penetration
2. Inhibit uncoating of virus in cells
3. Block primary transcription
4 Inhibit virus messenger RNA translation
5. Inhibit virus progeny assembly/maturation
6. Prevent release of mature virus or progeny from cells (i.e., confine)

As there have been a substantial number of neoplasms as well as glandular effects such as diabetes in this series, that must be considered in determining treatment.

Thus, appropriate treatment should be given in the initial infective stage. In poliomyelitis, it is very obvious that activity during the infective phase gravely exacerbates the subsequent pathology. This was also demonstrated for viral myocarditis in experiments with swimming mice. For picornaviruses, antiviral agents are not available, and therefore rest is mandatory. As shown in Groups 1 to 5, healing may be spontaneous or other sequelae may develop. In the rare case (e.g., F14) where a severe, reactive vasculitis occurs, steroids may have to be considered, but generally their administration is counterproductive. Again, as in Lord Horder's (1929) case, serological administration may be crucial, but these are very rare events. For those who go on to Groups 3 and 4, the support usually needed for specific organ dysfunction is required. Again, in very rare cases, either kidney or heart transplant has been required. No doubt, the earlier the diagnosis is made and effective treatment given, the less frequent would be the sequelae.

As in all areas of medicine, developments with excellent consequences, and sometimes adverse side effects, will occur. Until such time as more specific treatment is available, then empathy and support are undoubtedly potent agents in combating disease. It has been shown by many, and in varied ways, that isolation stress gravely interferes with immune resistance. During the forty years' experience briefly described in these chapters, it has been host response, sometimes linked with suitable medication, that has resulted in a satisfactory outcome. Empathy and kindness, in my opinion, have no adverse side effects and can be expected to synergize with whatever additional scientific treatment is available and will never be outmoded.

References

Adelstein and Donovan (1972). *MBMJ,* 1V:629.

Archard, L. (1991). In B.M. Hyde, J.A. Goldstein, and P.H. Levine (eds.), *Clinical and scientific basis of myalgic encephalomyelitis/chronic fatigue syndrome.* Ottawa: Nightingale Research Foundation.

Bakheit, A.M.O., Behan, P.O., Dinan, G.T., Gray, C.E., and O'Keene, V.G. (1992). Upregulation of 5-HT receptors in patients with PVFS. *British Medical Journal,* 304, 110-112.

Banatvala, J.E., et al. (1987). Evidence linking coxsackie B viruses with persistent infections in patients with chronic cardiac disease. *International Congress of Virology,* August.

Baron, S., Dianzari, F., and Stanton, G.J. (1982). General considerations of the interferon system. *Tex. Rep. Biol. Med.,* 41:1-12.

Beck, M.A., Shi, Q., Morris, V.C., and Levander, O.A. (1995). Rapid genomic evolution of a non-virulent Coxsackie B3 in selenium-deficient mice results in selection of identical virulent isolates.

Behan, P. (1991). In B.M. Hyde, J.A. Goldstein, and P.H. Levine (eds.), *The clinical and scientific basis of myalgic encephalomyelitis/chronic fatigue syndrome.* Ottawa: Nightingale Research Foundation.

Behan, P. et al. (1985). *Journal of Infection,* 10:211-222.

Bell, E.J. et al. (1988). Neurologic disorders. In M. Bendinelli and H. Friedman (eds.), *Coxsackieviruses: A general update.* New York: Plenum Press.

Ben-Nathan, D. *Life Sciences,* 48:1493-1500.

Ben-Nathan, D., Maestroni, G.J.M., Lustig, S., and Conti, A. (1994). The effects of melatonin on encephalitic arboviruses.

Ben-Nathan, D., Maestroni, G.J.M., Lustig, S., and Conti, A. (1995). Protective effects of melatonin in mice infected with encephalitis virus. *Archives of Virology,* 140:223-230.

Blumberg et al. (1967). Australian antigen. *Annals of Internal Medicine,* 66:924.

British Veterinary Journal (1988). 144:288.

Brunberg et al. *Archives of Neurology,* 30:304-306.

Burch, G.E. et al. (1967). Coxsackie B viral myocarditis and valvulitis identified in routine autopsy specimens by immunofluorescent techniques. Tulane University.

Butler et al. (1963). *Perinatal mortality.* Livingstone.

Caligiuri (1987). *Journal of Immunology,* 139:3306-3313.

Chandrobose et al. (1981). *Science,* 212:329-331.

Cooper et al. (1969). *American Journal of the Diseases of Children,* 118:18.

Costa, D.C. (1995). Single photon emission tomography (SPET) in M.E. patients, Research Workshop, Newcastle Research Group.

Curnen et al. (1961). *Yale Journal of Biological Medicine,* 24:959-963.

Demitrack, M.A., Daje, J.K., Straus, S.E., Laue-Lousia, et al. (1991). Evidence for impaired activation of the hypothalamic-pituitary-adrenal axis in patients with CFS. *Journal of Clinical Endocrine and Metabolism,* 73:1224-1234.

Dianzani, F. et al. (1988). The role of interferon in Picornavirus infections. In M. Bendinelli and H. Friedman (eds.), *Coxsackieviruses: A general update.* New York: Plenum Press.

Fedrick and Alberman (1982). *British Medical Journal,* ii:485.

Fleischmann, W.R. Jr. Interferon: Synergism and/or potentiation by interferons and other agents.

Friedman, H., et al. (1984). Virus interaction with immune defence system.

Fujinami and Oldstone (1986). Molecular mimicry and autoimmunity. In A. Szentivanyi and H. Friedman (eds.), *Viruses, Immunity and Immunodeficiency.* New York: Plenum Press.

Hamblin (1983). *British Medical Journal,* 287:85-88.

Heathfield et al. (1967). *Quarterly Journal of Medicine.*

Herberman, R.B. (1986). Viruses, cancer and immunity. In A. Szentivanyi and H. Friedman (eds.), *Viruses, Immunity and Immunodeficiency.* New York: Plenum Press.

Horder, T. (1929). A case of cerebral symptoms following vaccination. *Lancet,* June 22:1301.

Hyde, B., Biddle, R., and McNamara, T. (1991). Magnetic resonance in the diagnosis of M.E./CFS, a review. In B.M. Hyde, J.A. Goldstein, and P.H. Levine (eds.), *Clinical and scientific basis of myalgic encephalomyelitis/chronic fatigue syndrome.* Ottawa: Nightingale Research Foundation.

Hyde, B.M., Goldstein, J.A., and Levine, P.H. (eds.), *The clinical and scientific basis of myalgic encephalomyelitis/chronic fatigue syndrome.* Nightingale Research Foundation.

Jacobson et al. (1987). *Journal of Infection,* 14:103-111.

Jenkins, R. and Mowbray, J. (eds.) (1991). *Post-viral fatigue syndrome (myalgic encephalomyelitis).* New York: John Wiley.

Kandolf, R. (1988). The impact of recombinant DNA technology on the study of enterovirus heart disease. In M. Bendinelli and H. Friedman (eds.), *Coxsackieviruses: A general update.* New York: Plenum Press.

Khesin, Y.E. et al. (1978). Association between group G chromosomes, especially chromosome G21, and susceptibility of human cells to coxsackie B virus. *Bull. Exsp. Biol. Med.* (Russia).

Lerner, A.M. (1993). Repetitively negative changing T waves in patients with CFS/ME. *Chest,* 104.

Loria, R.M. (1986a). Coxsackievirus B, lipids and immunity as shared determinants in diabetes and atherosclerosis. In A. Szentivanyi and H. Friedman (eds.), *Viruses, Immunity and Immunodeficiency.* New York: Plenum Press.

Loria, R.M. (1986b). In A. Szentivanyi and H. Friedman (eds.), *Viruses, Immunity and Immunodeficiency.* New York: Plenum Press.

Loria, R.M. (1988). Host conditions affecting the course of coxsackie infections. In M. Bendinelli and H. Friedman (eds.), *Coxsackieviruses: A general update.* New York: Plenum Press.

Loria, R.M. (1992). *Archives of Virology,* 127:103-115.

Melnick, J. (ed.) (1974). *Progress in medical virology,* Volume 18. Basel: Karger, pp. 15-17.

Meltzer, H.Y., Flemming, R., and Robertson, A. (1983). The effect of buspirone on prolactin and growth hormone secretion in man. *Archives of General Psychiatry,* 40:1099-1102.

Mena, I. et al. (1991). Study of cerebrospinal perfusion by NeuroSPECT in patients with chronic fatigue syndrome, In B.M. Hyde, J.A. Goldstein, and P.H. Levine (eds.), *Clinical and scientific basis of myalgic encephalomyelitis/chronic fatigue syndrome.* Ottawa: Nightingale Research Foundation, p. 432.

Mumma, R.A. (1971). Paper presented to Federation of American Societies for Experimental Biology.

Oldham, R.K. (1984). Immunorestoration of immunodefiency by biological defence modifiers. University of British Columbia.

Peatfield, R.C. (1987). Basal ganglia damage and subcortical demential after possible insidious coxsackie virus encephalitis. *Acta Neurol. Scand.,* 76:340-345.

Plum (1956). Sensory loss with poliomyelitis. *Neurology,* 6:166-172.

Purves-Stewart. *Diseases of the nervous system,* p. 268.

Reiter, R.J. (1994). *Free radicals, melatonin, and cellular antioxidative defense mechanisms.* Stuttgart: Mattes Verlag.

Reyers, M.P. and Lerner, A.M. (1988). Myocarditis. In M. Bendinelli and H. Friedman (eds.), *Coxsackieviruses: A general update.* New York: Plenum Press.

Rosenberg et al. (1964). *Progress in CVS disease.*

Sadun, A.A. (1991) In B.M. Hyde, J.A. Goldstein, and P.H. Levine (eds.), *The clinical and scientific basis of myalgic encephalomyelitis/chronic fatigue syndrome.* Ottawa: Nightingale Research Foundation.

Sklarin, N.T., Chahinian, A.P., Peuer, E.J., Lahman, L.A., Szrajer, L., and Holland, J.F. (1988). Augmentation of activity of cis-diamminodichloroplatinum and mitimycin C by interferons in human malignant mesothelioma xenografts in nude mice. *Cancer Research,* 48(1):64-67.

Smith (1970). *American Heart Journal.*

Stewart, P.M., Maheshwaren, S., Griffith, J., and Li, J, et al. (1993). Pituitary imaging is essential for women with moderate hyperprolactinemia. *British Medical Journal,* 306:507-508.

Szentivanyi, A. and Friedman, H. (eds.) (1986). *Viruses, Immunity and Immunodeficiency.* New York: Plenum Press.

Toniolo, A., et al. (1984). The immune system in experimental coxcackievirus-B3 infection.

Trentin, J. (1986). In A. Szentivanyi and H. Friedman (eds.), *Viruses, Immunity and Immunodeficiency.* New York: Plenum Press, p. 153.

Williams et al. Serum fatty acid proportions are altered during the year following E.B. virus infection. *Lipids,* 23:981-988.

Winther, M.D. (1991). In B.M. Hyde, J.A. Goldstein, and P.H. Levine (eds.), *The clinical and scientific basis of myalgic encephalomyelitis/chronic fatigue syndrome.* Ottawa: Nightingale Research Foundation.

Woodruff, J.F. (1980). Viral myocarditis. *American Journal of Pathology,* 101: 427-429.

Index

Page numbers followed by the letter "i" indicate illustrations; those followed by the letter "t" indicate tables.